Health and Disease of American Indians North of Mexico

A Bibliography
1800–1969

COMPILERS

Mark V. Barrow, M.D., Ph.D.
Assistant Professor
Department of Medicine
Division of Cardiology
University of Florida
Gainesville, Florida

Jerry D. Niswander, D.D.S.
Chief, Human Genetics Branch
National Institute of Dental Research
National Institutes of Health
Bethesda, Maryland

Robert Fortuine, M.D., M.P.H.
Service Unit Director
Indian Health Service
United States Public Health Service
Fort Defiance, Arizona

Health and Disease of American Indians North of Mexico

A Bibliography
1800–1969

Compiled by
MARK V. BARROW, JERRY D. NISWANDER
AND
ROBERT FORTUINE

UNIVERSITY OF FLORIDA PRESS
GAINESVILLE · 1972

A University of Florida Press Book

Library of Congress Cataloging in Publication Data

Barrow, Mark V   1935–
  Health and disease of American Indians north of Mexico.
  1. Indians of North America—Health and hygiene—
Bibliography.   2. Indians of North America—Diseases—
Bibliography.   I. Niswander, Jerry D., 1930–
joint author.   II. Fortuine, Robert, 1934–   joint
author.   III.   Title.
Z6661.N67B3   016.61′09701   70–161004
ISBN 0–8130–0331–8

MANUFACTURED FOR THE PUBLISHER BY
ROSE PRINTING COMPANY
TALLAHASSEE, FLORIDA

MAJOR SOURCES FOR REFERENCES

a. *The Index Catalogue of the Library of the Surgeon General's Office,* beginning in 1880.

b. *US Bureau of American Ethnology Annual Reports,* beginning in 1882.

c. *Quarterly Cumulative Index Medicus,* beginning in 1916.

d. *Biological Abstracts,* beginning in 1926.

e. *Current List of Medical Literature,* beginning in 1941.

f. *Cumulated Index Medicus,* beginning in 1960.

g. *Library of Congress Catalog.*

h. *Arctic Bibliography.*

i. *The Health of the Eskimos: A Bibliography, 1857–1967*

j. *American Journal of Physical Anthropology,* vol 1–31.

k. *American Journal of Public Health,* vol 1–59.

l. *Canadian Journal of Public Health,* vol 1–60.

m. *Public Health Reports,* vol 1–84.

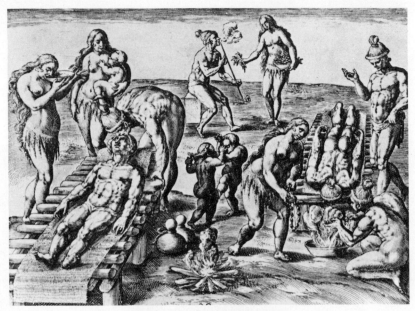

MODE OF TREATING THE SICK

"They put up a bench or platform of sufficient length and breadth for the patient . . . and lay the sick person upon it with his face up or down, according to the nature of his complaint; and, cutting into the skin of the forehead with a sharp shell, they suck out blood with their mouths, and spit it into an earthen vessel or a gourd bottle. Women who are suckling boys, or who are with child, come and drink this blood, particularly if it is that of a strong young man; as it is expected to make their milk better, and to render the children who have the benefit of it bolder and more energetic. For those who are laid on their faces, they prepare fumigations by throwing certain seeds on hot coals; the smoke being made to pass through the nose and mouth into all parts of the body, and thus to act as a vomit, or to overcome and expel the cause of the disease. They have a certain plant whose name has escaped me, which the Brazilians call *petum*, and the Spaniards *tapaco*. The leaves of this, carefully dried, they place in the wider part of a pipe; and setting them on fire, and putting the other end in their mouths, they inhale the smoke so strongly, that it comes out at their mouths and noses, and operates powerfully to expel the humors. In particular, they are extremely subject to the venereal disease, for curing which they have remedies of their own, supplied by nature." (Picture and description adapted from Charles E. Bennett, comp., *Settlement of Florida*, University of Florida Press, Gainesville, 1968.)

PREFACE

In 1562 the French sent a small garrison to what is now Northeast Florida. Settlers followed in 1564, among whom was Jacques Le Moyne de Morgues, a mapmaker. In 1565 the settlement was destroyed by the Spanish, but Le Moyne escaped and eventually ended up in London. There he wrote *Brevis Narratio* and executed a series of paintings about the Florida Indians. After Le Moyne's death, Theodore de Bry, a Flemish engraver, in 1588 purchased the pictures and narrative from Le Moyne's widow. The narrative and engravings of the pictures were printed with the second part of his *Grandes Voyages* under the title *Brevis Narratio corum quae in Florida Americae* (Frankfurt, 1591).

The illustration on the facing page depicts how the Florida Indians encountered by Le Moyne treated their sick. This bibliography is a compilation of modern medicine's attempt to treat and care for the North American Indian peoples. The contrast, to date, is not really so striking.

CONTENTS

I. GENERAL

   A. Bibliographical *items* 1–6

   B. Historical, Biographical, Autobiographical, and Personal Narratives *items* 7–82

II. STUDIES ON HEALTHY INDIVIDUALS

   A. Vital Statistics *items* 83–100

   B. Diet, Nutrition, and Growth *items* 101–132

   C. Physiology and Metabolism *items* 133–151

   D. Environmental Health *items* 152–157

III. INDIAN HEALTH AND DISEASE—GENERAL AND UNSPECIFIED

   A. Archeological Studies and Paleopathology *items* 158–221

   B. Diseases of Indians—Unspecified *items* 222–338

IV. HEALTH PROGRAMS FOR INDIANS

A. Health Surveys, Congressional Investigations, and Legislation   *items* 339–371

B. Statistical Publications and Annual Reports   *items* 372–434

C. General Health Programs and Services   *items* 435–647

V. INFECTIOUS AGENTS AND DISEASES

A. General and Unspecified   *items* 648–661
B. Partially Specified
   i. Upper and Lower Respiratory Infections   *items* 662–668
   ii. Gastrointestinal Infections   *items* 669–682
   iii. Central Nervous System Infections   *item* 683
   iv. Parasitic Infestations   *items* 684–690
C. Diseases Transmitted from Man to Man
   i. Viral
     a. General   *item* 691
     b. Polio   *items* 692–697
     c. Viral Meningitis   *item* 698
     d. Influenza   *items* 699–705
     e. Respiratory Viral Infections   *items* 706–707
     f. Hepatitis   *items* 708–712
     g. Enteroviruses   *items* 713–716
     h. Smallpox   *items* 717–726
     i. Measles   *items* 727–729
   ii. Trachoma   *items* 730–760
   iii. Bacterial (Excluding Tuberculosis)
     a. Bacterial Bronchitis and Pneumonias   *items* 761–763
     b. Streptococci Producing Scarlet Fever and Rheumatic Fever   *items* 764–768
     c. Nephritogenic Streptococci   *items* 769–777
     d. Staphylococci   *items* 778–779
     e. Salmonella-Shigella   *items* 780–784
     f. *Escherichia coli*   *items* 785–787
     g. Bacterial Meningitis   *item* 788

iv. Tuberculosis   *items* 789–926
v. Syphilis   *items* 927–933
vi. Amebiasis   *items* 934–939
vii. Helminth Infestations   *items* 940–942

D. Diseases Transmitted from Animals, Animal Products, or Soil to Man
  i. Zoonoses in General   *items* 943–948
  ii. Viral   *items* 949–951
  iii. Rickettsial   *item* 952
  iv. Bacterial
    a. Plague   *items* 953–959
    b. Tularemia   *items* 960–969
    c. Brucellosis   *item* 970
  v. Fungal   *items* 971–975
  vi. Malarial   *items* 976–979
  vii. Helminth Infestations
    a. Echinococcosis (Hydatid Disease)   *items* 980–991
    b. Trichinosis   *item* 992
    c. Diphyllobothriasis   *items* 993–994

VI. NEOPLASMS   *items* 995–1021

VII. MENTAL HEALTH AND PSYCHIATRIC DISORDERS

A. Mental Health and Hygiene   *items* 1022–1044

B. Alcoholism and Addiction   *items* 1045–1075

C. Suicide   *items* 1076–1079

D. Psychotic and Psychoneurotic Disorders   *items* 1080–1103

E. Stuttering   *items* 1104–1108

F. Other   *items* 1109–1125

VIII. PREGNANCY, CHILDBIRTH, AND GYNECOLOGICAL CONDITIONS   *items* 1126–1160

IX. CONGENITAL MALFORMATIONS

A. Inborn Errors of Metabolism   *items* 1161–1176

B. Other *items* 1177–1203

X. CHILD HEALTH AND DISEASES OF INFANCY OTHER THAN MALFORMATIONS *items* 1204–1225

XI. DISEASES OF THE INTEGUMENTARY SYSTEM *items* 1226–1230

XII. DISEASES OF THE MUSCULOSKELETAL SYSTEM *items* 1231–1255

XIII. DISEASES OF THE RESPIRATORY SYSTEM (CHRONIC) *items* 1256–1262

XIV. DISEASES OF THE CARDIOVASCULAR SYSTEM *items* 1263–1280

XV. DISEASES OF THE HEMATOPOIETIC SYSTEM INCLUDING HEMO-GLOBINOPATHIES *items* 1281–1292

XVI. DISEASES OF THE DIGESTIVE SYSTEM

A. Gallbladder Disease *items* 1293–1302
B. Other *items* 1303–1311

XVII. DISEASES OF THE ENDOCRINE SYSTEM

A. Diabetes Mellitus *items* 1312–1336
B. Other *items* 1337–1345

XVIII. DISEASES OF THE UROGENITAL SYSTEM *items* 1346–1347

XIX. DISEASES OF THE NERVOUS SYSTEM *items* 1348–1350

XX. DISEASES OF THE SENSE ORGANS

A. Eye
  i. Phlyctenular Keratoconjunctivitis *items* 1351–1357
  ii. Other *items* 1358–1370
B. Ear *items* 1371–1387

XXI. DENTAL STUDIES AND PROBLEMS *items* 1388–1460

CONTENTS

XXII. MISCELLANEOUS TOPICS

    A. Malnutrition and Vitamin Deficiencies *items* 1461–1470

    B. Trauma and Accidents *items* 1471–1476

    C. Other Miscellaneous Publications *items* 1477–1483

INDICES

    Author Index   p 119

    Subject Index   p 131

    Tribe Index   p 141

        Linguistic Stock of the Tribes Mentioned in the Tribe Index   p 145

INTRODUCTION

THIS BIBLIOGRAPHY lists publications about health and disease in American Indians north of Mexico, including Canadian and Arctic Indians. Since information regarding health of the Eskimos and Aleuts can be found in Robert Fortuine's *The Health of the Eskimos: A Bibliography, 1857–1967,* these groups are excluded. The bibliography has been compiled and arranged with the aim of providing public health personnel, clinicians, nurses, and medical scientists ready access to the medical literature on Indian health. Purposely omitted are publications about Indian beliefs regarding disease, the Indian medicine man, and various folk remedies and medicines. Anthropological studies not directly related to health, including demographic, linguistic, and social structure data are not included, since these subjects form topics in their own right. Statistical studies about blood types are also excluded unless they have a direct bearing on health and disease.

The major sources of the references for this bibliography are given on page v. By using these publications, additional references not previously listed in the major sources were frequently obtained

1

and used. Mrs. Ann Price, Information Office, Indian Health Service, also graciously furnished many published works of the United States Public Health Service not included in the major sources. To her we are grateful.

The National Institutes of Health Library and the National Library of Medicine were very helpful in locating and verifying older and hard to find articles. To them we express our sincere thanks.

Hopefully, this bibliography is comprehensive and thorough, although many narratives of early American travels describing health conditions in Indians prior to the nineteenth century are omitted. We do not believe this is a serious omission. The descriptions in these travels, by necessity, are generally vague and unhelpful, since they are subjective opinions written, for the most part, by nonmedically trained explorers.

As seen in the contents section, citations are arranged into 22 categories. The first section encompasses bibliographical and historical works, while studies on healthy individuals are covered in Section II. Then comes one of the largest divisions, Indian health and disease—unspecified (III), followed by comprehensive coverage of health programs for Indians (IV). Infectious agents and diseases (V) is the largest division (it includes infections involving multiple systems); infections of specific and single systems are listed in their respective categories. Neoplasms, mental health and psychiatric disorders, normal and abnormal pregnancy, congenital malformations, and diseases of infancy are given their own categories (VI–X). Sections XI through XX are divided by anatomical system, in accordance with the *International Classification of Diseases*. These sections are sometimes further subdivided by individual disease entities within each system if the number of articles appearing warrants such treatment. Section XXI lists references about dental problems and health, and Section XXII concludes the work with various miscellaneous topics.

Abbreviations of journals conform to those used in the *Index Medicus*, and the format follows the *AMA Style Book and Editorial Manual*. Publications are arranged chronologically by year and within each year alphabetically.

Three indices conclude this work. An author index is followed by an index arranged alphabetically by disease subject. A subject index was thought to be essential, since articles in the first four sections, in addition to discussing broad topics, frequently contain information on specific diseases. The subject index thus provides additional aid to researchers. The third index pertains to each tribe. The tribes listed are arranged alphabetically; a listing of the tribes by linguistic group, as given in C. Wissler's *The American Indian,* is included at the end of this index.

This bibliography is respectfully dedicated to our fellow Americans and brothers, the American Indian.

I. GENERAL

A. BIBLIOGRAPHICAL

1. *Bibliography on American Indian Medicine,* Smithsonian Inst, Bur of Amer Ethnology, 1957.

2. Driver, H.E., and Massey, W.C.: Comparative Studies of North American Indians, *Trans Amer Philosophical Soc* 47: 440–456, 1957.

3. Sturtevant, C.: *Bibliography on American Indian Medicine and Health,* Smithsonian Inst, Bur of Amer Ethnology, 1962.

4. Fortuine, R.: *The Health of the Eskimos: A Bibliography, 1857–1967,* Hanover, NH: Dartmouth Coll Lib, 1968.

5. *Indian Health in the US and Canada, January 1964–August 1968* (228 citations), Bibliography No. 20–68, US Dept of HEW, Natl Lib Med, 1968, pp 1–12.

6. *Indian Health in the US and Canada, Index Medicus, 1960–1963* (108 citations), US Public Health Serv, Natl Inst Health Lib, 1969.

5

B. HISTORICAL, BIOGRAPHICAL, AUTOBIOGRAPHICAL,
AND PERSONAL NARRATIVES

7. Josselyn, J.: *An Account of Two Voyages to New England,*
London, 1675.

8. LaHontan: *New Voyages to America,* 2 vol, London, 1703.

9. Rush, B.: An Oration Delivered February 4, 1774, Before the
American Philosophical Society, Held at Philadelphia, Con-
taining an Enquiry into the Natural History of Medicine
Among the Indians in North America, and a Comparative
View of Their Diseases and Remedies with Those of Civilized
Nations; Together with an Appendix Containing Proofs and
Illustrations, *Med Inquiry & Observations,* 1789, pp 5-6.

10. Parrish, J.: Account of a Fever Which Prevailed Among the
Indians on the Island of Nantucket in 1763-64, *Eclectic Rep*
1:364-366, 1811.

11. Hunter, J.D.: Remarks on Several Diseases Prevalent Among
the Western Indians, with Some Account of Their Remedies
and Modes of Treatment, *Amer Med Recorder* 5:408-417,
1822.

12. Hunter, J.D.: Remarks on the Diseases of the Females of
Several Indian Tribes West of the Mississippi, *New York Med
Phys J* 1:304-315, 1822.

13. Thomassen á Thuersink, E.J.: *Over de Ziekten en Derzelven
Behandling Door de Wilde Indianen in Noord-America,* Al-
gemeen Letterlieven Maandschrift Osten Deel, No. 5, Amster-
dam, 1824.

14. Wilkes, C.: *Narrative of the United States Exploring Expedition, 1835-1842,* Philadelphia, 1845, p 512.

15. Winder, W.: On Indian Diseases and Remedies; With a Re-
turn of Sick Treated at the Indian Establishment, Great
Manatoulin Island, Lake Huron, in 1841-42, *Brit Amer J* 1:
255-257, 1845-1846.

16. Romanowsky: Observations dans les Colonies Russes de
l'Amerique, *J Med de Russie,* No. 20, 1848.

17. Schoolcraft, H.R. (ed.): *Information Respecting the History,
Condition, and Prospects of the Indian Tribes of the United
States,* 6 vol, Philadelphia: Lippincott, Grambo & Co, 1852-
1857.

18. Andros, F.: "Medical Knowledge of the Indians: Historical and Statistical Information Respecting Indian Tribes of the US," in Schoolcraft, H.R. (ed.): *Information Respecting the History, Condition, and Prospects of the Indian Tribes of the United States*, vol 3, Philadelphia: Lippincott, Grambo & Co, 1853, pp 497–498.

19. DeForest, J.W.: *History of the Indians of Connecticut from the Earliest Known Period to 1850*, Hartford, Conn, 1853.

20. Evans, J.P.: Twelve Months' Practice in the Cherokee Nation, West, *Southern J Med Phys Sci* 2:12, 257, 317, 1854.

21. Moses: Medical Topography of Astoria, Oregon, *Amer J Med Serv* ns 29:32–46, 1855.

22. Suckley, G.: Report on the Fauna and Medical Topography of Washington Territory, *Trans Amer Med Ass* 19:183–217, 1857.

23. Lincoln, D.F.: Medical Notes upon the Aborigines of Alaska, *Boston Med Surg J* 83:353, 1870.

24. Wythe, W.T.: Medical Notes on Alaska, *Pacif Med Surg J* 4:337–342, 1870–1871.

25. Toner, J.M.: *Address Before the Rocky Mountain Medical Association, June 6th, 1877, Containing Some Observations on the Geological Age of the World, the Appearance of Animal Life upon the Globe, the Antiquity of Man, and the Archaeological Remains of Extinct Races Found on the American Continent, with Views of the Origin and Practices of Medicine Among Civilized Races, More Especially the North American Indians*, Washington, DC, 1877.

26. Toner, J.M.: Some Points in the Practice of Medicine Among the North American Indians, with Incidental Reference to the Antiquity of the Office of the Physician, *Virginia Med Mon* 4:334–340, 1877.

27. Jones, J.: Explorations and Researches Concerning the Destruction of the Aboriginal Inhabitants of America by Various Diseases Such as Syphilis, Matlazahuatl, Pestilence, Malarial Fever, and Smallpox, *N Orleans Med Surg J* 5:926–941, 1877–1878.

28. McClenachan, H.M.: The Practice of Medicine Among the Indians, *Med Surg Reporter* 44:338–341, 1881.

29. Mathews, P.W.: Notes on Diseases Among the Indians Fre-

quenting York Factory, Hudson's Bay, *Canad Med Surg J* 13:449–466, 1884–1885.

30. Thorworth, J.F.: Indian Practice on the Northern Coast of California, *St Joseph Med Herald* 4:130, 1886.

31. Whitney, W.F.: Notes on the Anomalies, Injuries, and Diseases of the Native Races of North America, *Rep Peabody Mus* 3 (Rep 18–19):433–448, 1886.

32. Neave, J.L.: An Agency Doctor's Experiences Among Frontier Indians, *Cincinnati Med J* 9:875, 1894; 10:611–616, 1895; and 11:17–23, 1896.

33. Hefferman, W.T.: Medicine Among the Yumas, *Calif Med J* 17:135–140, 1896.

34. Thwaites, R.G. (ed.): *Jesuit Relations and Allied Documents, 1601–1791*, 74 vol, Cleveland: A. H. Clark Co, 1896–1901.

35. Thwaites, R.G. (ed.): *Early Western Travels, 1748–1846*, 32 vol, Cleveland: A. H. Clark Co, 1904–1907.

36. Duxrury, J.: Difficulties in Practice Amongst the Indians, *W Canad Med J* 1:403–415, 1907.

37. Moody, C.S.: A Physician Among the Indians, *Amer J Clin Med* 14:161, 310, 1907.

38. Ferguson, F.D.: Medical Practice Among the Indians, *Amer J Clin Med* 16:997–1000, 1909.

39. Grinnell, F.: Some Reminiscences of Indian Practice, *Calif State Med J* 7:174–177, 1909.

40. Williams, H.V.: The Epidemic of the Indians of New England, 1616–1620, with Remarks on Native American Infections, *Bull Hopkins Hosp* 20:340–349 (Nov) 1909.

41. Neave, J.L.: Medical Practice Among the Indians, *Amer J Clin Med* 16:1325, 1909; and 17:25, 1910.

42. Krulish, E.: Some Surgical Experiences Among Indians of Alaska, *JAMA* 64:1748, 1915.

43. Cobb, C.M.: Medical Practice Among the New England Indians and Early Settlers, *Boston Med Surg J* 177:97, 1917.

44. Shaw, W.F.: Medical Experiences Among Kwquithlik Indians Along Discovery Passage, B.C., *Canad Med Ass J* 13:657–659, 1923.

45. Grenfell, W.T.: Medicine in the Sub-Arctic, Mary Scott New-

bold Lecture, Lecture 12, *Trans Coll Physicians Phila* 52:73–95, 1930.

46. Jones, H.: Historical Medicine; Indian and White Man, *Med J Rec* 134:297, 1931.

47. Sticker, G.: Epidemics Brought to the New World by White Conquerors, *Rev Hig Tuberc* 24:78–83, 1931.

48. Stone, E.: Surgery Among the North American Indians, *Amer J Surg* 13:579–584, 1931.

49. Simmons, J.S.: Influence of Epidemic Disease on Early History of the Western Hemisphere, *Milit Surg* 71:133–143, 1932.

50. Stone, E.: Medicine Among the Iroquois, *Ann Med Hist* 6:529–539, 1934.

51. Cook, S.F.: Diseases of Indians of Lower California in the Eighteenth Century (Translation of Jesuit Document), *Calif Western Med* 43:432–434, 1935.

52. Loree, D.R.: Notes on Alaskan Medical History, *Northwest Med* 34:262–268, 1935.

53. Urquhart, J.A.: The Most Northerly Practice in Canada, *Canad Med Ass J* 33:193–196 (Aug) 1935.

54. Ashburn, P.M.: How Disease Came with the White Man: Stories of Early Medical Milestones in America, *Hygeia* 14:514, 636, 1936.

55. Townsend, J.G.: Medical and Health Work Among the North American Indians, *Health Officer* 2:350–352, 1937.

56. Wissler, C.: *Indian Cavalcade, or, Life on the Oldtime Indian Reservations*, New York: Sheridan House, 1938.

57. Aberle, S.B.D.; Watkins, J.H.; and Pitney, E.H.: Vital History of San Juan Pueblo, *Hum Biol* 12:141–187, 1940.

58. Aronson, J.D.: The History of Disease Among the Natives of Alaska, *Trans Coll Physicians Phila* ns 8:27–46, 1940.

59. Yule, R.F.: A Year with the Indians, *Manitoba Med Rev* 22:246–247, 1942.

60. Hrdlička, A.: *Alaska Diary, 1926–1931*, Lancaster, Pa: Jacques Cattell Press, 1943, p 414.

61. Beaugrand-Champagne, A.: Les Maladies et la Médecine des Anciens Iroquois, *Cah Dix* 9:227–242, 1944.

62. Corrigan, R.S.C.: Medical Practice Among the Bush Indians

of Northern Manitoba, *Canad Med Ass J* 54:220–223 (March) 1946.

63. Aronson, J.D.: The History of Disease Among the Natives of Alaska, *Alaska's Health* 5 (No. 3–7) 1947.

64. Larsell, O.: Medical Aspects of the Lewis and Clark Expedition (1804–1806), *Surg Gynec Obstet* 85:663–669 (Nov) 1947.

65. Moorman, L.J.: Pioneer Medicine in the Southwest, *Bull Hist Med* 21:795–810 (Sept–Oct) 1947.

66. Gordan, B.L.: *Medicine Throughout Antiquity*, Philadelphia: F. A. Davis Co, 1949.

67. Falconer, W.L.: The Charles Camsell Indian Hospital, *Arctic Circle* 3:17–18 (Feb–March) 1950.

68. Adams, W.R.: Aboriginal American Medicine and Surgery, *Proc Indiana Acad Sci* 61:49–53, 1952.

69. Ward, K.A.: Arctic Interlude, *Canad Med Ass J* 67:292–298 (Oct) 1952.

70. Larson, J.A.: Medicine Among the Indians, *Quart Bull Northwestern U Med School* 27:246–249, 1953.

71. Schaefer, O.: Eingeborenen Medizin bei Indianern und Eskimos im Äusserten Norden Kanada, *München Med Wschr* 99: 1833–1835, 1957.

72. Crockett, B.N.: Health Conditions in the Indian Territory to 1890, *Chronicles of Oklahoma* 36:21–39, 1958.

73. MD for Indians Taps Rich Medical, Human Experience, *House Physician* 2:1–3 (March) 1962.

74. Romanowsky, P., and Frankenhauser, E.: Five Years of Medical Observations in the Colonies of the Russian-American Company, Part I and Part II, *Alaska Med* 4:33–37, 62–65, 1962.

75. Romig, J.H.: Medical Practice in Western Alaska Around 1900, *Alaska Med* 4:85–87, 1963.

76. Van Duzen, J.L.: Medical Practice on the Navajo Reservation, *J Amer Med Wom Ass* 19:558–560, 1964.

77. Kartchner, M.M.: Two Years with the American Indians, *Med Times* 93:124A–142A, 1965.

78. Kartchner, M.M.: Two Years with the American Indians, *Resident Physician* 11:70–85 (April) 1965.

79. Graham-Cumming, G.: Health of the Original Canadians, 1867–1967, *Med Serv J Canada* 23:115–166, 1967.

80. Navajo Doctor, *Baylor Med* (Feb) 1967, pp 1–6.

81. Swan, R.: The History of Medicine in Canada, *Med Hist* 12: 42–45 (Jan) 1968.

82. Thompson, R.R.: After Two Years in Alaska with the USPHS, *Alaska Med* 10:191–192, 1968.

II. STUDIES ON HEALTHY INDIVIDUALS

A. VITAL STATISTICS

83. Flower, W.H.: The American Races, *Brit Med J* 1:549–577, 1880.

84. Yarrow, H.C.: Medical Facts Relating to the Zuni Indian of New Mexico, *Rocky Mountain Med Rev* 1:193–194, 1880–1881.

85. The Vital Statistics of an Apache Indian Community, *Publ Amer Statis Ass* ns 3:426–428, 1892–1893.

86. Borden, W.C.: The Vital Statistics of an Apache Indian Community, *Boston Med Surg J* 129:5–10, 1893.

87. Moody, C.I.: The Nez Perce Indians, *Amer J Clin Med* 18: 406–507, 1911.

88. Sniffen, M.K., and Carrington, T.S.: *The Indians of the Yukon and Tanana Valleys, Alaska*, Indian Rights Ass, 2nd Ser, No. 9B, Philadelphia, 1914, p 35.

89. *Indian Population in the United States and Alaska, 1910*, US Dept of Commerce, Bur of Census, 1915.

90. *Indians of North Carolina*, 63rd Congress, 3rd Session, US Senate, Doc 677, 1915.

91. Krogman, W.M.: Vital Data on the Population of the Seminole Indians of Florida and Oklahoma, *Hum Biol* 7:335–349, 1935.

92. Watkins, J.H.; Pitney, E.H.; and Aberle, S.B.D.: Vital Statistics of the Pueblo Indians, *Amer J Public Health* 29:753–760 (July) 1939.

93. Lorimer, F.: "Observations on the Trend of Indian Population in the United States," in La Farge, O. (ed.): *Changing Indian,* Norman: U of Okla Press, 1942, pp 11–18.

94. Hrdlička, A.: *The Aleutian and Commander Islands and Their Inhabitants,* Philadelphia: Wistar Inst, 1945, p 172.

95. Hanna, B.L.; Dahlberg, A.A.; and Strandskov, H.H.: Preliminary Study of Population History of Pima Indians, *Amer J Hum Genet* 5:377–388 (Dec) 1953.

96. Jones, C.F.: Demographic Patterns in the Papago Indian Village of Chuichu, Arizona, *Hum Biol* 25:191–202 (Sept) 1953.

97. White, C.B.: *An Outline of San Carlos Apache Culture,* US Public Health Serv, Div of Indian Health, Phoenix, Ariz, 1958.

98. Kluckhohn, C. (ed.): *The Navaho,* rev ed, New York: Doubleday and Co, 1962.

99. *Indians of Arizona,* US Dept of Interior, Bur of Indian Affairs, 1966.

100. Gurunanjappa, B.S.: Life Tables for Alaskan Natives, *Public Health Rep* 84:65–69 (Jan) 1969.

B. Diet, Nutrition, and Growth

101. Wakefield, E.G., and Dellinger, S.C.: Diet of Bluff Dwellers of Ozark Mountains and Its Skeletal Effects, *Ann Int Med* 9:1412–1418, 1936.

102. Carpenter, T.M., and Steggerda, M.: The Food of the Present-day Navajo Indians of New Mexico and Arizona, *J Nutr* 18: 287–305, 1939.

103. Price, W.A.: Light from Primitive Races on Relation of Nutrition to Individual and National Development, *J Amer Dent Ass* 26:938–948, 1939.

104. Moore, P.E., et al: Medical Survey of Nutrition Among Northern Manitoba Indians, *Canad Med Ass J* 54:223–233, 1946.

105. Duncan, A.C.: Diet and Disease in the Subarctic, *Lancet* 253:919–921, 1947.

106. Vivian, R.P., et al: The Nutrition and Health of the James Bay Indian, *Canad Med Ass J* 59:505-518 (Dec) 1948.

107. Pett, L.B.: "Nutrition Survey Methods as Applied to Pacific Coast Canadian Indians," in *Proc Pacif Sci Conf*, vol 7, New Zealand, 1949.

108. Sinclair, H.M.: The Diet of Canadian Indians and Eskimos, *Proc Nutr Soc* 12:69-82, 1953.

109. *Some Observations on the Nutritional Status of Alaskan Natives*, US Public Health Serv, Arctic Health Res Center, Anchorage, Alaska, 1954.

110. Vavich, M.G.; Kemmerer, A.R.; and Hirsch, J.S.: The Nutritional Status of Papago Indian Children, *J Nutr* 54:121-132 (Sept) 1954.

111. Darby, W.J., et al: Dietary Background and Nutrition of the Navajo, *J Nutr* 60 (suppl 2):1-85 (Oct) 1956.

112. Hursch, L.M.: Nutrition Survey of the Alaskan Eskimo and Indian, abstracted, *Sci in Alaska*, Proc 9th Alaskan Sci Conf (1958), AAAS, Alaska Div, 1960, pp 131-132.

113. Bosley, B.: Nutrition in the Indian Program, *J Amer Diet Ass* 35:905-909 (Sept) 1959.

114. Hesse, F.G.: A Dietary Study of the Pima Indian, *Amer J Clin Nutr* 7:532-537 (Sept-Oct) 1959.

115. Coffin, R.: Changing Food Habits Among Alaska Natives, *Alaska Med* 2:5-7, 1960.

116. Newman, M.T.: Adaptations in the Physique of American Aborigines to Nutritional Factors, *Hum Biol* 32:288-313 (Sept) 1960.

117. Stefansson, V.: "Food and Food Habits in Alaska and Northern Canada," in Galdston, I. (ed.): *Human Nutrition: Historic and Scientific*, New York: International Universities Press, 1960, pp 23-60.

118. Yearsley, E.: Nutrition in the Canadian North, *Northern Affairs Bull* 7:30-33, 1960.

119. Talcott, M.I., and Schuck, C.: Diets and Nutritional Status of Adolescent Indian Girls in Boarding Schools of the Dakotas, abstracted, *Proc S Dakota Sci* 40:245-246, 1961.

120. Newman, M.T.: Ecology and Nutritional Stress in Man, *Amer Anthrop* 64:22–34, 1962.

121. Schuck, C.; Wenberg, B.G.; and Talcott, M.I.: Nutritive Value of the Boarding School Diets of Sioux Indian Children, abstracted, *Fed Proc* 21:387, 1962.

122. Scott, E.M., and Heller, C.A.: "Nutrition of a Northern Population," Doc 18 in *Conf on Med and Public Health in the Arctic and Antarctic,* WHO, Geneva, 1962, p 26.

123. Mayberry, R.H., and Lindeman, R.D.: A Survey of Chronic Disease and Diet in Seminole Indians in Oklahoma, *Amer J Clin Nutr* 13:127–134 (Sept) 1963.

124. *Fort Belknap Indian Reservation Nutrition Survey: A Report by the Interdepartmental Committee on Nutrition for National Defense and the Division of Indian Health,* US Public Health Serv, Div of Indian Health, 1964.

125. Heller, C.A.: The Diet of Some Alaskan Eskimos and Indians, *J Amer Diet Ass* 45:425–428 (Nov) 1964.

126. Longman, D.P.: Working with Pueblo Indians in New Mexico, *J Amer Diet Ass* 47:470–473 (Dec) 1965.

127. Wenberg, B.G.; Boedeker, M.T.; and Schuck, C.: Observations on Growth and Development of Adolescent Sioux Indian Girls: Nutritive Value of Diets in Indian Boarding Schools in the Dakotas, *J Amer Diet Ass* 46:96–102 (Feb) 1965.

128. Heller, C.A., and Scott, E.M.: *The Alaska Dietary Survey, 1956–1961, Anchorage, Alaska,* US Public Health Serv, Publ 999-AH2, 1967.

129. Scott, E.M., and Heller, C.A.: Nutrition in the Arctic, *Arch Environ Health* 17:603–608 (Oct) 1968.

130. Wuerffel, S.: Nutrition Work Among the Sioux, *Illinois Diet Ass Bull* 34 (Spring) 1968.

131. *Conference on Nutrition, Growth, and Development of North American Indian Children, May 19–22, 1969, Norman, Oklahoma* (sponsored by Natl Inst of Child Health and Hum Develop; Indian Health Serv Com on Indian Health; and Amer Acad of Pediat), 1969.

132. Payne, W.: Food for First Citizens, *Civil Rights Dig* (Fall) 1969, pp 1–4.

C. PHYSIOLOGY AND METABOLISM

133. Boteler, W.C.: Peculiarities of American Indians from Physiological and Pathological Standpoint, *Maryland Med J* 7:54–58, 1880–1881.

134. Shaw, M.M.: The Basal Metabolism of Some American Indian Girls, *J Amer Diet Ass* 9:120–123, 1933.

135. Dunham, E.C., et al: Physical Status of 219 Pueblo Indian Children, *Amer J Dis Child* 53:739–749, 1937.

136. Crile, G.W., and Quiring, D.P.: Indian and Eskimo Metabolisms, *J Nutr* 18:361–368, 1939.

137. Coffey, M.F.: "A Comparative Study of Young Eskimo and Indian Males with Acclimatized White Males," in *Conf on Cold Injury*, Trans of Third Macy Conf (Feb 22, 23, 24, and 25, 1954), Fort Churchill, Manitoba, 1955, pp 100–116.

138. Hayman, C.R., and Kester, E.R.: *A Comparative Study of Alaska Natives and US Indians*, Juneau, Alaska (Sept) 1957.

139. Adams, T., and Covino, B.G.: Racial Variations to a Standardized Cold Stress, *J Appl Physiol* 12:9–12 (Jan) 1958.

140. Andersen, K.L., et al: Physical Fitness of Arctic Indians, *J Appl Physiol* 15:645–648 (July) 1960.

141. Elsner, R.W.; Andersen, K.L.; and Hermansen, L.: Thermal and Metabolic Responses of Arctic Indians to Moderate Cold Exposure at the End of Winter, *J Appl Physiol* 15:659–661 (July) 1960.

142. Elsner, R.W.; Nelms, J.D.; and Irving, L.: Circulation of Heat to the Hands of Arctic Indians, *J Appl Physiol* 15:662–666 (July) 1960.

143. Irving, L., et al: Metabolism and Temperature of Arctic Indian Men During a Cold Night, *J Appl Physiol* 15:635–644 (July) 1960.

144. Hart, J.S.: *Comparison of Responses to Cold in Eskimos with Those of Caucasians, Alakulufe Indians, and Australian Aborigines*, US Army Med Res Lab, Rep 474, 1961, p 51.

145. Milan, F.A.; Evonuk, E.; and Hannon, J.P.: Comparative Study of Thermoregulation in Eskimos, Indians, and US Soldiers, abstracted, *Sci in Alaska*, Proc 12th Alaskan Sci Conf (1961), AAAS, Alaska Div, 1962, p 191.

146. Hammel, H.T.: Effect of Race on Response to Cold, *Fed Proc* 22 (No. 3, pt 1):795–800, 1963.

147. Milan, F.A.; Hannon, J.P.; and Evonuk, E.: Temperature Regulations of Eskimos, Indians, and Caucasians in a Bath Calorimeter, *J Appl Physiol* 18:378–382 (March) 1963.

148. Eagan, C.J., and Evonuk, E.: Retention of Resistance to Cooling by Alaskan Natives Living in a Temperate Climate, abstracted, *Fed Proc* 23 (No. 2, pt 1):367, 1964.

149. Lutwak, L., et al: Effects of High Dietary Calcium and Phosphorus on Calcium, Phosphorus, Nitrogen, and Fat Metabolism in Children, *Amer J Clin Nutr* 14:76–85 (Feb) 1964.

150. Cumming, G.R.: Current Levels of Fitness, *Canad Med Ass J* 96:868–882 (March) 1967.

151. Irving, L.: Adaptations of Native Populations to Cold, *Arch Environ Health* 17:592–594 (Oct) 1968.

D. ENVIRONMENTAL HEALTH

152. Durham, W.F., et al: Insecticide Content of Diet and Body Fat of Alaskan Natives, *Science* 134:1880–1881 (Dec) 1961.

153. Hanson, W.C., and Palmer, H.E.: The Accumulation of Fallout Cesium 137 in Northern Alaskan Natives, *Trans N Amer Wildlife Conf* 29:215–225, 1964.

154. Hanson, W.C.; Palmer, H.E.; and Griffin, B.I.: *Second Survey of Radioactivity in Northern Alaskan Natives and Their Foods, Summer 1963*, Hanford Atomic Products Operation, HW 80500 (Jan 15) 1964, pp 191–194.

155. Hanson, W.C., and Palmer, H.E.: Seasonal Cycle of Cs-137 in Some Alaskan Natives and Animals, *Health Phys* 11:1401–1406, 1965.

156. Palmer, H.E., et al: Radioactivity Measurements in Alaskan Natives, 1962–1964, *Science* 147:620–621 (Feb) 1965.

157. Chance, N.A.: Implications of Environmental Stress; Strategies of Developmental Change in the North, *Arch Environ Health* 17:571–577 (Oct) 1968.

III. INDIAN HEALTH AND DISEASE— GENERAL AND UNSPECIFIED

A. Archeological Studies and Paleopathology

158. Hirsch, A.: *Handbook of Geographical and Historical Pathology*, London: New Sydenham Soc, 1883.

159. Moodie, R.L.: The Antiquity of Potts' Disease and Other Spinal Lesions; Primitive Treatment, *Surg Clin* 4:619–627, 1920.

160. Moodie, R.L.: Surgery and Disease Among the Pre-Columbian Indians of North America, *Surg Clin* 4:1091–1102, 1920.

161. Means, H.J.: Roentgenological Study of Skeletal Remains of Prehistoric Mound Builder Indians of Ohio, *Amer J Roentgen* 13:359–367, 1925.

162. Bentzen, R.C.: Dental Conditions Among Mimbres People of Southwestern United States Previous to Year 600 A.D.; Original Study of Teeth and Jaws from Series of Skeletons Unearthed by Jenks Expedition, *Dent Cosmos* 71:1068–1073, 1929.

163. Leigh, R.W.: Dental Pathology of Aboriginal California, *Dent Cosmos* 71:756–767, 1929.

164. Moodie, R.L.: Deafness Among Ancient Californian Indians, *Bull Southern Calif Acad Sci* 28 (pt 3):46–49, 1929.

165. Bödecker, C.F.: Defects in Enamel of Teeth of Ancient American Indians, *J Dent Res* 10:313–322, 1930.

166. Moodie, R.L.: Teeth, Jaws, and Palates in Pre-Pueblo Indians from New Mexico, *Pacif Dent Gaz* 38:127–145, 1930.

167. Moodie, R.L.: What Bad Teeth Did to a Pre-historic Indian, *Hygeia* 8:551–552, 1930.

168. Tello, J.C., and Williams, H.V.: An Ancient Syphilitic Skull, *Ann Med Hist* 2:515–529, 1930.

169. Denninger, H.S.: Cervical Ribs: A Prehistoric Example, *Amer J Phys Anthrop* 16:211–213, 1931.

170. Denninger, H.S.: Osteitis Fibrosa in a Skeleton of a Prehistoric American Indian, *Arch Path* 11:939–947, 1931.

171. Fisher, A.K.; Kuhm, H.W.; and Adami, G.C.: Dental Pa-

thology of Prehistoric Indians of Wisconsin, *Bull Public Mus, City of Milwaukee* 10:329–334, 1931.

172. Moodie, R.L.: Prehistoric Maxillofacial Diseases, *Biol Med (Milano)* 7:373–376, 1931.

173. Congdon, R.T.: Spondylolisthesis and Vertebral Anomalies in Skeletons of American Aborigines, with Clinical Notes on Spondylolisthesis, *J Bone Joint Surg [Amer]* 14:511–524, 1932.

174. Rihan, H.Y.: Dental and Orthodontic Observations on 289 Adult and 53 Immature Skulls from Pecos, NM, *Intl J Orthodont* 18:708–712, 1932.

175. Ritchie, W.A., and Warren, S.L.: The Occurrence of Multiple Bony Lesions Suggesting Myeloma in the Skeleton of a Pre-Columbian Indian, *Amer J Roentgen* 28:622–628, 1932.

176. Williams, H.V.: The Origin and Antiquity of Syphilis: The Evidence from Diseased Bones, *Arch Path* 13:779–814, 931–983, 1932.

177. Hrdlička, A.: Seven Prehistoric American Skulls with Complete Absence of External Auditory Meatus, *Amer J Phys Anthrop* 17:355–377 (Jan–March) 1933.

178. Denninger, H.S.: Prehistoric Syphilitic Lesions (An Example from North America), *Southwest Med* 19:202–204, 1935.

179. Prehistoric American Indians Suffered from Syphilis, editorial, *Science* 83 (suppl):(April 7) 1936.

180. Williams, H.V.: The Origin of Syphilis: Evidence from Diseased Bones, *Arch Derm Syph* 33:783–787 (May) 1936.

181. Canavan, M.M.: Enostoses Within the Calvarium; Survey of Skulls in Warren Museum of Harvard University Medical School, *Arch Neurol Psychiat* 38:1240–1242, 1937.

182. Rice, C.E.: Ophthalmologic Indications of Disease: Study of Ancient Skulls in National Museum, *Amer J Ophthal* 20:1045–1046, 1937.

183. Denninger, H.S.: Syphilis of a Pueblo Skull Before 1350, *Arch Path* 26:724–727, 1938.

184. Halton, W.L., and Shands, A.R., Jr.: Evidence of Syphilis in Mound Builder's Bones: Gross Pathologic Study, *Arch Path* 25:228–242, 1938.

185. Malattie Pre-Colombiane fra gli Indiani d'America, *Minerva Med* 31 (pt 1):360–364, 1940.

186. Hrdlička, A.: Diseases of and Artifacts in Skulls and Bones from Kodiak Island, *Smithsonian Miscellaneous Collections* 101 (No. 4) 1941.

187. Williams, G.D.; Ritchie, W.A.; and Titterington, P.E.: Multiple Bony Lesions Suggesting Myeloma in a Pre-Columbian Indian Aged 10 Years, *Amer J Roentgen* 46:351–355, 1941.

188. Rabkin, S.: Dental Conditions Among Prehistoric Indians of Northern Alabama, *J Dent Res* 21:211–222, 1942.

189. Rabkin, S.: Dental Conditions Among the Prehistoric Indians of Kentucky, *J Dent Res* 22:355–366, 1943.

190. Cressman, L.S., and Larsell, O.: Probable Osteomyelitis in an Indian Skeleton; Case, *Western J Surg* 53:332–335, 1945.

191. Webb, G.B., and Stallings, W.S., Jr.: Pre-Columbian Tuberculosis, *Trans Amer Clin Climat Ass* 59:1–18, 1948.

192. "Clinical" Observations on American Archeology, *Trans Ass Amer Physicians* 63:29–34, 1950.

193. Courville, C.B.: Cranial Injuries Among Early Indians of California, *Bull Los Angeles Neurol Soc* 17:137–162, 1952.

194. Ritchie, W.A.: Paleopathologic Evidence Suggesting Pre-Columbian Tuberculosis in New York State, *Amer J Phys Anthrop* ns 10:305–317 (Sept) 1952.

195. Goldstein, M.S.: Some Vital Statistics Based on Skeletal Material, *Hum Biol* 25:3–12 (Feb) 1953.

196. Goldstein, M.S.: Skeletal Pathology of Early Indians in Texas, *Amer J Phys Anthrop* 15:229–307 (Sept) 1957.

197. Snyder, R.G.: Hyperdontia in Prehistoric Southwestern Indians, *Southwest J Anthrop* 16:492–502, 1960.

198. Morse, D.: Prehistoric Tuberculosis in America, *Amer Rev Resp Dis* 83:489–504 (April) 1961.

199. St. Hoyme, L.E., and Bass, W.M.: *Human Skeletal Remains from the Tollifero and Clarksville Site, Virginia*, Smithsonian Inst, Bur of Amer Ethnology, Bull 182, 1962, pp 329–400.

200. Chapman, F.H.: The Incidence and Age Distribution of Osteoarthritis in an Archaic American Indian Population, *Proc Indiana Acad Sci* 73:64–66, 1963.

201. Neumann, H.W.: A Preliminary Study in the Paleopathology of an Archaic American Indian Population, *Proc Indiana Acad Sci* 74:87–89, 1964.

202. Gregg, J.B.; Steele, J.P.; and Holzhueter, A.M.: Roentgeno-graphic Valuation of Temporal Bones from South Dakota Indian Burials, *Amer J Phys Anthrop* 23:51–61 (March) 1965.

203. Holzhueter, A.M.; Gregg, J.B.; and Clifford, S.: A Search for Stapes Foot-plate Fixation in an Indian Population, Prehistoric and Historic, *Amer J Phys Anthrop* 23:35–40 (March) 1965.

204. Jarcho, S.: Anomaly of the Vertebral Column (Klippel-Feil Syndrome) in American Aborigines, *JAMA* 193:843–844 (Sept) 1965.

205. Steele, J.P.: Paleopathology in the Dakotas, *S Dakota J Med* 18:17–29, 1965.

206. Wells, C.: *Bones, Bodies, and Disease; Evidence of Disease and Abnormality in Early Man,* New York: Praeger, 1965.

207. Beck, C.W., and Mulvaney, W.P.: Apatitic Urinary Calculi from Early American Indians, *JAMA* 195:1044–1045 (March) 1966.

208. Jarcho, S. (ed.): *Human Paleopathology,* New Haven, Conn: Yale U Press, 1966.

209. Bennett, K.A.: Craniostenosis: A Review of the Etiology and a Report of New Cases, *Amer J Phys Anthrop* 27:1–9 (July) 1967.

210. Brothwell, D.R., and Sandison, A.T. (eds.): *Diseases in Antiquity: A Survey of the Diseases, Injuries, and Surgery of Early Populations,* Springfield, Ill: Charles C Thomas, 1967.

211. Kelln, E.E.; McMichael, E.V.; and Zimmermann, B.: A Seven-teenth-Century Mandibular Tumor in a North American Indian, *Oral Surg* 23:78–81 (Jan) 1967.

212. Discovery of Prehistoric Cemetery Reveals Ohio Indians with Arthritis and Bad Teeth, *J Amer Dent Ass* 77:792–793 (Oct) 1968.

213. Koritzer, R.T.: Apparent Tooth Preparation in a Middle Mississippi Indian Culture, *J Dent Res* 47:839–844 (Sept–Oct) 1968.

214. Lester, C.W., and Shapiro, H.E.: Vertebral Arch Defects in the Lumbar Vertebrae of Pre-Historic American Eskimos—A Study of Skeletons in the American Museum of Natural History, Chiefly from Point Hope, Alaska, *Amer J Phys Anthrop* 28:43–48 (Jan) 1968.

215. McHenry, H.: Transverse Lines in Long Bones of Prehistoric California Indians, *Amer J Phys Anthrop* 29:1–17 (July) 1968.

216. Goldstein, M.S.: Human Paleopathology and Some Diseases in Living Primitive Societies, *Amer J Phys Anthrop* 31:285–293 (Nov) 1969.

217. Mehta, J.D.: A Comparative Study of the Dentition of the Shell Mound Indians of Alabama, *Alabama J Med Sci* 6:208–212 (April) 1969.

217A. Mehta, J.D.: A Study of Attrition and Malocclusion in the Dentition of Shell Mound Indians of Alabama, *Amer J Orthodont* 55:306–307 (March) 1969.

218. Moore, J.G.; Fry, G.F.; and Englebert, E.: Thorny-headed Worm Infection in North American Prehistoric Man, *Science* 163:1324–1325 (March) 1969.

219. Post, P.W., et al: Histological and Histochemical Examination of American Indian Scalps, Mummies, and a Shrunken Head, *Amer J Phys Anthrop* 30:269–293 (March) 1969.

220. St. Hoyme, L.E.: On the Origin of New World Paleopathology, *Amer J Phys Anthrop* 31:295–302 (Nov) 1969.

221. Stewart, T.D., et al: Lesions of the Frontal Bone in American Indians, *Amer J Phys Anthrop* 30:89–109 (Jan) 1969.

B. DISEASES OF INDIANS—UNSPECIFIED

222. Darling, D.: Indian Diseases and Remedies, *Boston Med Surg J* 34:9–13, 1846.

223. Stratton, T.: Contribution to an Account of the Diseases of the North American Indians, *Edinburgh Med Surg J* 71:269–283, 1849.

224. Glisan, R.: Climate and Diseases of Oregon, *Amer J Med Sci* 20:73–82, 1865.

225. Kneeland, T.: On Some Causes Tending to Promote the Extinction of the Aborigines of America, *Trans Amer Med Ass* 15:253, 1865.

226. Smart, C.: Notes on the Tonto Apaches, *Rep Smithsonian Inst, 1867*, Washington, DC, 1868, pp 417–419.

227. Andrews, E.: Military Surgery Among the Apache Indians, *Chicago Med Exam* 19:599–601, 1869.

228. Williamson, T.: The Diseases of the Dakota Indians, *Northwestern Med Surg J* 4:410–419, 1874.

229. Grinnell, F.: Indian Questions from a Medical Standpoint, *Cincinnati Lancet Observer* 21:157–169, 1878.

230. Meek, E.G.: Physical Condition of the Aborigines, with an Account of Their Practice of Medicine, *Illinois Indiana Med Surg J* 2:310–318, 1878.

231. Andros, F.: The Medicine and Surgery of the Winnebago and Dakota Indians, *JAMA* 1:116–118, 1883.

232. Treon, F.: Medical Work Among the Sioux Indians, *JAMA* 10:224–227, 1888.

233. Yarrow, H.C.: Medical Facts Relating to the Zuni Indian of New Mexico, *Rocky Mountain Med J* 1:193–194, 1888.

234. Woodruff, C.E.: Diseases of Northern California Indians, *Med Rec* 36:104–106, 1891.

235. (*Ninth*) *Annual Report of the Bureau of American Ethnology, 1887–1888,* Smithsonian Inst, Bur of Amer Ethnology, 1892, pp 39–40, 460.

236. Holder, A.B.: Papers on Diseases Among the Indians, *Med Rec* 42:117, 329, 357, 1892.

237. (*Fifteenth*) *Annual Report of the Bureau of American Ethnology, 1893–1894,* Smithsonian Inst, Bur of Amer Ethnology, 1897, pp 191–199.

238. Ranke, K.: Über die Sehschärfe der Indianer, *Centralblatt f Antrop usw* 2:342, 1897.

239. (*Seventeenth*) *Annual Report of the Bureau of American Ethnology, 1895–1896,* Smithsonian Inst, Bur of Amer Ethnology, 1898, pp 168, 173, 218, 219, 223, 289, 347, 362.

240. Benedict, A.L.: A Medical View of the American Indians of the Northeast, *Med Age* 19:767–771, 1901.

241. Lake, A.D.: The Civilized Indian, His Physical Characteristics, and Some of His Diseases, *NY Med J* 75:406–409, 1902.

242. Millard, T.F.: The Passing of the American Indian, *Forum* 34:466–480, 1903.

243. Hrdlička, A.: Diseases of the Indians, More Especially of the Southwest United States and Northern Mexico, *Washington Med Ann* 4:372–394, 1905.

244. Fehlinger, H.: Krankheiten der Nordamerikanischen Indianer, *Naturwiss Wschr* 21:697–699, 1906.

245. Hrdlička, A.: *Physiological and Medical Observations*, Smithsonian Inst, Bur of Amer Ethnology, Bull 34, 1908, pp 172–219.

246. Hodge, F.W.: *Handbook of American Indians North of Mexico*, Smithsonian Inst, Bur of Amer Ethnology, Bull 30, 1911, p 540.

247. Krulish, E.: Report upon Diseases Found Among the Indians of Southeast Alaska, *Public Health Rep* 29:1300, 1914.

248. Eastman, C.A.: The Indians' Health Problem, *Popular Sci Mon* 86:49–54, 1915.

249. Hrdlička, A.: Some Diseases Prevalent Among Indians of the Southwest and Their Treatment, *Med World* 33:305–310, 1915.

250. Geare, R.I.: Diseases of Indians of the Southwest and Their Treatment, *N Orleans Med Surg J* 68:359–370, 1915–1916.

251. Hrdlička, A.: The Vanishing Indian, *Science* 46:266, 1917.

252. Fleming, H.C.: Medical Observations Made on Zuni Indians, *Nation's Health* 5:506–508, 1923.

253. Fleming, H.C.: *Medical Observations on the Zuni Indians*, Contributions from the Mus of the Amer Indian, New York City, Heye Foundation, vol 7 (No. 2) 1924.

254. Emerson, H.: Health of American Indians, *JAMA* 88:424, 1927.

255. Guthrie, M.C.: Health of American Indians, *JAMA* 88:1198, 1927.

256. Health of American Indians, editorial, *JAMA* 88:104–105, 1927.

257. (*Forty-fourth*) *Annual Report of Bureau of American Ethnology, 1926–1927*, Smithsonian Inst, Bur of Amer Ethnology, 1928, pp 266, 335.

258. Brooks, H.: The Medicine of the American Indian, *Bull NY Acad Med* 5:509–537, 1929.

259. Guthrie, M.C.: The Health of the American Indian, *Public Health Rep* 44:945–957, 1929.

260. Brailsford, A.M.: Medical Service in Alaska, *Milit Surgeon* 67:585–591, 1930.

261. Hoffman, F.L.: Are the Indians Dying Out? *Amer J Public Health* 20:609–614, 1930.

262. Michael, L.F.: United States Indian Service, Department of Medicine and Surgery, Cheyenne River Sioux Indians, Cheyenne Agency, South Dakota, *J Lancet* 51:363–368, 381–385, 1931.

263. Hrdlička, A.: Disease, Medicine, and Surgery Among the American Aborigines, *JAMA* 99:1661–1666, 1932.

264. Stone, E.: *Medicine Among the American Indians*, New York: Hafner Pub Co, 1932.

265. Brooks, H.: The Medicine of the American Indian, *J Lab Clin Med* 19:1–23 (Oct) 1933.

266. Collier, J.: Indian Health, *Proc Conf State Prov Health Author N Amer* 48:56–62, 1933.

267. Darby, G.E.: Indian Medicine in British Columbia, *Canad Med Ass J* 28:433–438, 1933.

268. Hancock, J.C.: Diseases Among the Indians, *Southwest J Med Surg* 17:126–129, 1933.

269. Dickie, W.M.: Indian Health in California, *Proc Conf State Prov Health Author N Amer* 51:110–113, 1936.

270. Indian Mortality in California, *Week Bull Calif Dept Public Health* 15:85, 1936.

271. Marshall, L.R.: Health Studies Among the Indians, *Trained Nurse* 97:41–46, 1936.

272. Tillim, S.J.: Health Among the Navajos, *Southwest Med* 20: 355, 388, 432, 1936.

273. Tillim, S.J.: Medical Annals of Arizona, *Southwest Med* 20: 273, 310, 355, 388, 452, 1936.

274. Wissler, C.: Distribution of Deaths Among American Indians, *Hum Biol* 8:223–231, 1936.

275. Wissler, C.: The Effect of Civilization upon the Length of Life of the American Indian, *Sci Mon* 43:5–13, 1936.

276. Cook, S.F.: *The Extent and Significance of Disease Among*

the Indians of Baja California, 1697–1773, Berkeley: U of Calif Press, 1937, p 39.

277. Salsbury, C.G.: Disease Incidence Among the Navajos, *Southwest Med* 21:230–233 (July) 1937.

278. Townsend, J.G.: Diseases and the Indian, *Sci Mon* 48 (Dec) 1938.

279. Wissler, C.: The American Indian, *Ciba Symposia* 1:3–36, 1939.

280. Will They Give It Back to the Indians? *Penn Med J* 44:63–68, 1940–1941.

281. Walkin, F.: Social and Medical Aspects of Manitouwapah Indians, *Manitoba Med Rev* 21:157–160, 1941.

282. Report of the Committee on Indian Affairs, *Proc Conf State Prov Health Author N Amer* 56:87–90, 1941; and 57:234–245, 1942.

283. Townsend, J.G.: "Indian Health: Past, Present, and Future," in La Farge, O. (ed.): *Changing Indian,* Norman: U of Okla Press, 1942, pp 28–41.

284. Leighton, A.H., and Leighton, D.C.: *The Navajo Door,* Cambridge: Harvard U Press, 1944.

285. Winters, S.R.: Health for the Indian, *Hygeia* 22:680, 1944.

286. Ashburn, F.D.: *The Ranks of Death,* New York: Coward-McCann, 1947.

287. Barnett, H.E., et al: Medical Conditions in Alaska, *JAMA* 135:500–510 (Oct) 1947.

288. Salsbury, C.G.: Incidence of Certain Diseases Among the Navajos, *Arizona Med* 4:29–31 (Nov) 1947.

289. Woods, O.T.: Health Among the Navajo Indians, *JAMA* 135:981–983 (Dec) 1947.

290. Van Wart, A.F.: Indians of the Maritime Provinces; Diseases and Native Cures, *Canad Med Ass J* 59:573–577 (Dec) 1948.

291. Foard, F.T.: The Health of the American Indians, *Amer J Public Health* 39:1403–1406 (Nov) 1949.

292. Joseph, A.; Spicer, R.B.; and Chesky, J.: *The Desert People,* Chicago: U of Chicago Press, 1949, pp 177–184.

293. Moorman, L.J.: Health of the Navajo-Hopi Indians; General

Report of the American Medical Association, *JAMA* 139:370–376 (Feb) 1949.

294. Salsbury, C.G.: White Medicine for the Red Man, *Mod Hosp* 74:51–53, 1950.

295. *Proceedings of the First National Conference on Indian Health, Association on American Indian Affairs,* New York (June) 1953.

296. Kraus, B.S., and Jones, M.: *Indian Health in Arizona,* U of Ariz, Dept of Anthrop, Second Ann Rep of the Bur of Ethnic Res, 1954.

297. Hadley, J.N.: Health Conditions Among Navajo Indians, *Public Health Rep* 70:831–836 (Sept) 1955.

298. Slotnick, H.E., and Salisbury, L.H. (eds.): *Science in Alaska, 1955 and 1956* (combination of 16 articles), Proc 6th and 7th Alaskan Sci Conf, AAAS, Alaska Div, 1955, 1956.

299. Detal, C.S.: *Surgical Experience in Selected Areas of the US,* US Public Health Serv, monograph 38 (No. 473):45, 1956.

300. Adair, J.; Deuschle, K.W.; and McDermott, W.: Patterns of Health and Diseases Among the Navajos, *Ann Amer Acad Polit Sci* 311:80–94, 1957.

301. *Proceedings of the Second National Conference on Indian Health Held by the Association on American Indian Affairs,* New York (April) 1957.

302. Hildes, J.A., et al: Old Crow—A Healthy Indian Community, *Canad Med Ass J* 81:837–841 (Nov 15) 1959.

303. Schaefer, O.: Medical Observations and Problems in the Canadian Arctic, *Canad Med Ass J* 81:248–253, 386–393 (Aug) 1959.

304. Alaska—Frontier for Health Services, *Public Health Rep* 75:877–912 (Oct) 1960.

305. Gottmann, A.W.: A Report of One Hundred Three Autopsies on Alaskan Natives, *Arch Path* 70:117–124 (July) 1960.

306. Lemon, F.R.: Health Problems of the Navajos in Monument Valley, Utah, *Public Health Rep* 75:1055–1061 (Nov) 1960.

307. McNeilly, M.M.: *The Wonderful Years,* New York: Exposition Press, 1961.

308. Young, R.W.: *Navajo Yearbook,* Report VIII: *1951–1961,* Window Rock, Ariz: Navajo Agency, 1961.

309. "Health of the Navajo," in *The Navajo Yearbook, 1951–61*, US Public Health Serv, Div of Indian Health, 1962.

310. Best, E.W.R.: Disease and Death in Canada's North, editorial, *Med Serv J Canada* 19:775–777, 1963.

311. Jenness, D.: *The Indians of Canada*, Natl Mus of Canada, Anthrop Ser 15, Bull 65, Ottawa: Queen's Printer, 1963.

312. Kester, F.E.: "Alaska's Population as Seen Through Its Death Rates," in *Sci in Alaska*, Proc 13th Alaskan Sci Conf (1962), AAAS, Alaska Div, 1963, pp 194–209.

313. *Trends in Indian Health and Health Services, 1961 and 1962*, US Public Health Serv, Div of Indian Health, 1963.

314. Willis, J.S.: Disease and Death in Canada's North, *Med Serv J Canada* 19:747–768, 1963.

315. Hesse, F.G.: Incidence of Disease in the Navajo Indian, *Arch Path* 77:553 (May) 1964.

316. Kravetz, R.E.: Disease Distribution in Southwestern American Indians: Analysis of 211 Autopsies, *Arizona Med* 21:628 (Sept) 1964.

317. Men and Medicine, *Med Sci* 15:52, 1964.

318. *Proceedings of the Third National Conference on Indian Health—Auspices of the National Committee on Indian Health*, Ass on Amer Indian Affairs, New York (Nov) 1964.

319. Fahy, A., and Muschenheim, C.: Third National Conference on American Indian Health, *JAMA* 194:1093–1096 (Dec) 1965.

320. Geography and Health, *Canad Med Ass J* 93:1322–1323 (Dec) 1965.

321. Muskakoo, V.E.: Health and Living Conditions of the American Indian, *Zdravookhr Ross Fed* 10:36–39 (July) 1966.

322. *Proceedings of the First Joint Meeting of the Clinical Society and Commissioned Officers Association of the United States Public Health Service*, Baltimore, Md (May) 1966.

323. *Proceedings of the Fourth National Conference on Indian Health*, Ass on Amer Indian Affairs, Natl Com on Indian Health, New York (Nov) 1966.

324. Sievers, M.L.: Disease Patterns Among Southwestern Indians, *Public Health Rep* 12:1075 (Dec) 1966.

325. Autopsies and Southwestern American Indians, editorial, *JAMA* 201:55 (July) 1967.

326. Health Problems of the American Indian, *Currents in Public Health* 7:1–4, 1967.

327. Porvaznik, J.: Traditional Navajo Medicine, *General Practitioner* 34:179–182, 1967.

328. *Proceedings of the Second Joint Meeting of the Clinical Society and Commissioned Officers Association of the United States Public Health Service,* Atlanta, Ga (May) 1967.

329. Reichenbach, D.: Autopsy Incidence of Diseases Among Southwestern American Indians, *Arch Path* 84:81 (July) 1967.

330. *Biomedical Challenges Presented by the American Indian,* WHO, Proc Special Session of the 7th Meet of Pan Amer Health Org, Publ 165, 1968.

331. *Current Project Summaries—Published Monograph Abstracts,* US Public Health Serv, Indian Health Serv, Health Program Systems Center, Tucson, Ariz (Sept) 1968.

332. Fleshman, J.K.: Health of Alaska Native Children, *Alaska Med* 10:39–42, 1968.

333. Neel, J.V.: "The American Indian in the International Biological Program," in *Biomedical Challenges Presented by the American Indian,* WHO, Pan Amer Health Org, Publ 165, 1968, pp 47–58.

334. *Proceedings of the Third Joint Meeting of the Clinical Society and Commissioned Officers Association of the United States Public Health Service,* San Francisco, Calif (March) 1968.

335. *Indian Record* (special health issue), US Dept of Interior, Bur of Indian Affairs (June) 1968, p 8.

336. *Proceedings of the Fifth National Conference on Indian Health,* Ass on Amer Indian Affairs, Natl Com on Indian Health, New York (March) 1969.

337. *Proceedings of the Fourth Joint Meeting of the Clinical Society and Commissioned Officers Association of the United States Public Health Service,* Boston (June) 1969.

338. Proceedings of the Fourth National Conference on Indian Health, III: Environmental Factors, *Arch Environ Health* 19:429–458 (Sept) 1969.

IV.   HEALTH   PROGRAMS   FOR   INDIANS

A.   Health Surveys, Congressional Investigations,
and Legislation

339. *Condition of the Indian Tribes* (rep of the Joint Special Com appointed under joint resolution on March 3, 1865), US Congress, 1867.

340. *A Bill to Create the Office of Medical Inspector for the United States Indian Service*, 47th Congress, 1st Session, US Senate, Doc 929 (Jan 24) 1882.

341. *Survey of Conditions of the Indians in the United States*, 47th Congress, 1st Session, US Senate, Doc 929 (Jan 24) 1882.

342. Emmons, G.T.: *Conditions and Needs of the Natives of Alaska* (message from the President of the US, transmitting a rep on the condition and needs of the natives of Alaska), 58th Congress, 3rd Session, US Senate, Doc 106, 1905.

343. *Survey of Conditions of the Indians in the United States*, Part 7: *South Dakota*, 71st Congress, 2nd Session, US Senate, Com on Indian Affairs, 1930, pp 2753–3013.

344. *Survey of Conditions of the Indians in the United States*, Part 23: *Montana*, 72nd Congress, 1st Session, US Senate, Com on Indian Affairs, 1932, pp 12311–12975.

345. Hamlin, H.: Health Survey of Seminole Indians, *Yale J Biol Med* 6:155–177, 1933.

346. *Survey of Conditions of the Indians in the United States*, Part 30: *Minnesota and North Dakota*, 73rd Congress, US Senate, Com on Indian Affairs, 1934, pp 16145–16510.

347. *Survey of Conditions of Indians in the United States*, Part 36: *Alaska*, 74th Congress, 2nd Session, US Senate, Subcom of Com on Indian Affairs, 1939, pp 19, 703–719.

348. Cohen, F.S.: *Handbook of Federal Indian Law*, US Dept of Interior, 1941, p 455.

349. Innis, H.A.; Wherrett, G.J.; and Moore, A.: Survey of Health Conditions and Medical and Hospital Services in the Northwest Territories, *Canad J Econ Polit Sci* (Feb) 1945, p 35.

350. *US Commission on Organization of the Executive Branch*

of the Government, Rep of the Com on Indian Affairs (Oct) 1948.

351. Braasch, W.F.; Branton, B.J.; and Chesley, A.J.: Survey of Medical Care Among the Upper Midwest Indians, *JAMA* 139:220–226 (Jan) 1949.

352. *Transferring the Maintenance and Operations of Hospital and Health Facilities for Indians to the PHS: Report to Accompany HR 303,* 83rd Congress, 1st Session, House, Com on Interior and Insular Affairs, House Rep 870, 1953.

353. Indian Health Services Transferred to PHS, *Public Health Rep* 69:866 (Sept) 1954.

354. Indian Medical Service Transfer to Public Health Service, editorial, *Amer J Public Health* 44:1449, 1461–1462 (Dec) 1954.

355. Moore, P.E.: Health for Indians and Eskimos, *Canad Geogr J* 48:216–221, 1954.

356. *Transfer of Indian Hospitals and Health Facilities to Public Health Service,* 83rd Congress, 2nd Session, US Senate, Com on Interior and Insular Affairs, Hearings on HR 303 (May 28–29) 1954.

357. *Transferring Maintenance and Operation of Hospital and Health Facilities for Indians to the Public Health Service,* 83rd Congress, 2nd Session, US Senate, Com on Interior and Insular Affairs, Senate Rep 1530, 1954.

358. Cameron, C.M., Jr.: Cherokee Indian Health Survey, *Public Health Rep* 71:1086–1088 (Nov) 1956.

359. Moore, P.E.: Medical Care of Canada's Indians and Eskimos, *Canad J Public Health* 47:227–233 (June) 1956.

360. *Construction of Indian Hospitals,* 85th Congress, House, Com on Interstate and Foreign Commerce, 1st Session on HR 2021 and HR 2380 (April 9) 1957.

361. *Amending the Act of August 5, 1954 (Which Transferred Indian Health to the PHS),* 85th Congress, 2nd Session, US Senate, Com on Labor and Public Welfare, Senate Rep 1876, 1958.

362. *Indian Sanitation Facilities,* US Congress, House, Com on Interstate and Foreign Commerce, 1959.

363. *Indian Sanitation Facilities: Report to Accompany S56,* US

Congress, House, Com on Interstate and Foreign Commerce, 1959.

364. *Declaring the Sense of Congress on the Closing of Indian Hospitals*, 86th Congress, 2nd Session, House, Com on Interior and Insular Affairs, House Rep 1205, 1960.

365. *A Review of the Indian Health Program*, 88th Congress, 1st Session, House, Com on Interior and Insular Affairs (May 23) 1963.

366. *A Review of the Indian Health Program*, 90th Congress, 1st Session, House, Com on Interior and Insular Affairs, 1967.

367. *Hearings Before the Special Subcommittee on Indian Education of the Committee on Labor and Public Welfare*, Part 5: *May 24, 1968, Portland, Ore, and Oct 1, 1968, Washington, DC*, 90th Congress, 1st and 2nd Sessions, 1969, pp 1907-2371.

368. *Hearings Before the Special Subcommittee on Indian Education of the Committee on Labor and Public Welfare*, Part 4: *April 16, 1968, Pine Ridge, SD*, 90th Congress, 1st and 2nd Sessions, 1969, p 1229.

369. *Hearings Before the Special Subcommittee on Indian Education of the Committee on Labor and Public Welfare*, Part 1: *Dec 14-15, 1967, Washington, DC, and Jan 4, 1968, San Francisco, Calif*, 90th Congress, 1st and 2nd Sessions, 1969, pp 1-535.

370. *Hearings Before the Special Subcommittee on Indian Education of the Committee on Labor and Public Welfare*, Part 3: *March 30, 1968, Flagstaff, Ariz*, 90th Congress, 1st and 2nd Sessions, 1969, pp 989-1228.

371. *Hearings Before the Special Subcommittee on Indian Education of the Committee on Labor and Public Welfare*, Part 2: *Feb 19, 1968, Twin Oaks, Calif*, 90th Congress, 1st and 2nd Sessions, 1969, pp 537-988.

B. STATISTICAL PUBLICATIONS AND ANNUAL REPORTS

372. *Annual Reports of the Commissioner of Indian Affairs to the Secretary of the Interior for the Years 1869-70 to 1882-3*, US Dept of Interior, 1870-1883.

373. *Consolidated Reports of Sick and Wounded in the US Indian*

Service, US Bur of Indian Affairs, Com on Indian Affairs, 1879–1895.

374. Cogswell, W.F.: *Report of the Commissioner of Indian Affairs,* US Dept of Interior, 1932–1934 (also *Proc Conf State Prov Health Author N Amer* 47:111, 1932; 48:62, 1933; and 49:43, 1934).

375. Townsend, J.G.: Commissioner's Annual Report, 1939, *Proc Conf State Prov Health Author N Amer* 55:107–114, 1940.

376. *Annual Report for the Fiscal Year Ended March 31, 1946–48,* Canad Dept of Natl Health and Welfare, Ottawa: King's Printer, 1946–1949.

377. *Illness Among Indians, 1955,* US Public Health Serv, Div of Indian Health (1st ed after transfer of Indian Health to Public Health Serv).

378. *Annual Discharge Summary,* US Public Health Serv, Div of Indian Health, 1957 (1st in series).

379. *Illness Among Indians, 1957–1959,* US Public Health Serv, Div of Indian Health (2nd in series).

380. *Indians on Federal Reservations in the US—A Digest: Billings Area,* US Public Health Serv, Div of Indian Health, Publ 615, pt 2, 1958.

381. *Indians on Federal Reservations in the US—A Digest: Portland Area,* US Public Health Serv, Div of Indian Health, Publ 615, pt 1, 1958.

382. *Indians on Federal Reservations in the US—A Digest: Aberdeen Area,* US Public Health Serv, Div of Indian Health, Publ 615, pt 3, 1959.

383. *Annual Discharge Summary,* US Public Health Serv, Div of Indian Health, 1960 (2nd in series; none issued in 1958 or 1959).

384. *Illness Among Indians, 1960,* US Public Health Serv, Div of Indian Health (3rd in series).

385. *Indians on Federal Reservations in the US—A Digest: Albuquerque Area,* US Public Health Serv, Div of Indian Health, Publ 615, pt 4, 1960.

386. *Indians on Federal Reservations in the US—A Digest: Oklahoma City Area and Florida,* US Public Health Serv, Div of Indian Health, Publ 615, pt 5, 1960.

387. *Annual Discharge Summary,* US Public Health Serv, Div of Indian Health, 1961 (3rd in series).

388. *Indian Health Highlights,* 5th ed, US Public Health Serv, Div of Indian Health, 1961 (1st ed after transfer of Indian Health to the Public Health Serv).

389. *Indians on Federal Reservations in the US—A Digest: Phoenix Area,* US Public Health Serv, Div of Indian Health, Publ 615, pt 6, 1961.

390. *Illness Among Indians, 1961–1962,* US Public Health Serv, Div of Indian Health (called *Ann Statis Rev* also; 4th in series).

391. *Illness Among Indians, 1962,* US Public Health Serv, Div of Indian Health (5th in series).

392. *Annual Discharge Summary,* US Public Health Serv, Div of Indian Health, 1962–1963 (4th in series).

393. *Annual Statistical Review, Hospital and Medical Services, Fiscal Year 1963,* US Public Health Serv, Div of Indian Health, 1963.

394. *Eskimos, Indians, and Aleuts of Alaska—A Digest,* US Public Health Serv, Div of Indian Health, Publ 615, pt 7, 1963.

395. *Illness Among Indians, 1963,* US Public Health Serv, Div of Indian Health (6th in series).

396. *Annual Discharge Summary: Fiscal Year 1964,* US Public Health Serv, Div of Indian Health (5th in series).

397. *Illness Among Indians, 1964,* US Public Health Serv, Div of Indian Health (7th in series).

398. *Indian Health Highlights,* 6th ed, US Public Health Serv, Div of Indian Health, 1964.

399. *Annual Discharge Summary: Fiscal Year 1965,* US Public Health Serv, Div of Indian Health (6th in series).

400. *Discharge Summary and Analysis, Fiscal Years 1962 and 1963, Public Health Service, Indian and Alaska Native Hospital and Contract Hospitals,* US Public Health Serv, Div of Indian Health, 1965.

401. *Illness Among Indians, 1965,* US Public Health Serv, Div of Indian Health (8th in series).

402. *Annual Discharge Summary, 1966,* US Public Health Serv, Div of Indian Health (7th and last in series; after this ed,

combined with *Illness Among Indians* to become *Ann Statis Rev*).

403. *Annual Report—Fiscal Year 1966,* US Public Health Serv, Div of Indian Health, 1966.

404. *Illness Among Indians, 1966,* US Public Health Serv, Div of Indian Health (9th and last in series; after this ed, combined with *Annual Discharge Summary* to become *Ann Statis Rev*).

405. *Indian Health Highlights—1966,* 7th ed, US Public Health Serv, Div of Indian Health (June) 1966.

406. *Annual Statistical Review, Hospital and Medical Services, Fiscal Year 1967: Indian and Alaska Native Hospitals,* US Public Health Serv, Div of Indian Health (Dec) 1967.

407. *Division Summary, Morbidity and Mortality, 1967,* US Public Health Serv, Div of Indian Health, 1967.

408. *1967 Indian Vital Statistics—Washington,* US Public Health Serv, Div of Indian Health, Health Program Systems Center, Tucson, Ariz (Dec) 1967.

409. *To the First Americans, First Annual Report on the Indian Health Program of the US Public Health Service,* US Public Health Serv, Div of Indian Health, 1967.

410. *Annual Report: Fiscal Year 1968—Nursing Services Branch,* US Public Health Serv, Health Serv and Mental Health Administration, Indian Health Serv, 1968.

411. *Indian Health Highlights, 1968,* 8th ed, US Public Health Serv, Div of Indian Health (charts only; after this ed, becomes *Indian Health Trends and Serv*).

412. *1967 Indian Vital Statistics—Colorado,* US Public Health Serv, Div of Indian Health, Health Program Systems Center, Tucson, Ariz (Oct) 1968.

413. *1967 Indian Vital Statistics—Florida,* US Public Health Serv, Div of Indian Health, Health Program Systems Center, Tucson, Ariz (Oct) 1968.

414. *1967 Indian Vital Statistics—Idaho,* US Public Health Serv, Div of Indian Health, Health Program Systems Center, Tucson, Ariz (Oct) 1968.

415. *1967 Indian Vital Statistics—Iowa,* US Public Health Serv, Div of Indian Health, Health Program Systems Center, Tucson, Ariz (Oct) 1968.

416. *1967 Indian Vital Statistics—Kansas,* US Public Health Serv, Div of Indian Health, Health Program Systems Center, Tucson, Ariz (Sept) 1968.

417. *1967 Indian Vital Statistics—Mississippi,* US Public Health Serv, Div of Indian Health, Health Program Systems Center, Tucson, Ariz (Oct) 1968.

418. *1967 Indian Vital Statistics—Nebraska,* US Public Health Serv, Div of Indian Health, Health Program Systems Center, Tucson, Ariz (Sept) 1968.

419. *1967 Indian Vital Statistics—Nevada,* US Public Health Serv, Div of Indian Health, Health Program Systems Center, Tucson, Ariz (April) 1968.

420. *1967 Indian Vital Statistics—New Mexico,* US Public Health Serv, Div of Indian Health, Health Program Systems Center, Tucson, Ariz (May) 1968.

421. *1967 Indian Vital Statistics—North Carolina,* US Public Health Serv, Health Serv and Mental Health Administration, Indian Health Serv, Health Program Systems Center, Tucson, Ariz (Nov) 1968.

422. *1967 Indian Vital Statistics—Oregon,* US Public Health Serv, Health Serv and Mental Health Administration, Indian Health Serv, Health Program Systems Center, Tucson, Ariz (Dec) 1968.

423. *1967 Indian Vital Statistics—Utah,* US Public Health Serv, Health Serv and Mental Health Administration, Indian Health Serv, Health Program Systems Center, Tucson, Ariz (Nov) 1968.

424. *1967 Indian Vital Statistics—Wisconsin,* US Public Health Serv, Div of Indian Health, Health Program Systems Center, Tucson, Ariz (June) 1968.

425. *To the First Americans, Second Annual Report on the Indian Health Program of the US Public Health Service,* US Public Health Serv, Div of Indian Health, Publ 1580, 1968.

426. *Annual Statistical Review, Hospital and Medical Services, Fiscal Year 1968: Illness Among Indians and Alaska Natives, Calendar Year 1967,* US Public Health Serv, Health Serv and Mental Health Administration, Indian Health Serv (March) 1969.

427. *Indian Health Trends and Services—1969 Edition,* US Public Health Serv, Health Serv and Mental Health Administration, Indian Health Serv (March) 1969.

428. *1967 Indian Vital Statistics—Arizona,* US Public Health Serv, Health Serv and Mental Health Administration, Indian Health Serv, Health Program Systems Center, Tucson, Ariz (Jan) 1969.

429. *1967 Indian Vital Statistics—North Dakota,* US Public Health Serv, Health Serv and Mental Health Administration, Indian Health Serv, Health Program Systems Center, Tucson, Ariz (Jan) 1969.

430. *1967 Indian Vital Statistics—Oklahoma,* US Public Health Serv, Health Serv and Mental Health Administration, Indian Health Serv, Health Program Systems Center, Tucson, Ariz (Jan) 1969.

431. *1967 Indian Vital Statistics—South Dakota,* US Public Health Serv, Health Serv and Mental Health Administration, Indian Health Serv, Health Program Systems Center, Tucson, Ariz (May) 1969.

432. *To the First Americans, Third Annual Report on the Indian Health Program,* US Public Health Serv, Health Serv and Mental Health Administration, Indian Health Serv, Publ 1580, 1969.

433. *Annual Statistical Review, Hospital and Medical Services for American Indians and Alaska Natives, Fiscal Year 1969,* US Public Health Serv, Health Serv and Mental Health Administration, Indian Health Serv (Feb) 1970.

434. *Annual Statistical Review, Hospital and Medical Services for American Indians and Alaska Natives, Fiscal Year 1970,* US Public Health Serv, Health Serv and Mental Health Administration, Indian Health Serv (Feb) 1971.

C. GENERAL HEALTH PROGRAMS AND SERVICES

435. Pitcher, Z.: "Medicine," in Schoolcraft, H.R. (ed.): *Information Respecting the History, Condition, and Prospects of the Indian Tribes of the United States,* vol 4, Philadelphia: Lippincott, Grambo and Co, 1856.

436. Dowler, B.: Researches into the Sanitary Condition and Vital Statistics of Barbarians, *N Orleans Med Surg J* 14:335–352, 1857.

437. Kneeland, T.: Remarks on the Social and Sanitary Condition of the Onondago Indians, *Amer Med Times* 9:4–6, 1864.

438. Waldron, M.M.: The Indian School in Relation to Health, *Sanitarian* 36:303–310, 1896.

439. Benedict, A.L.: The American Aborigines from a Hygienic Standpoint, *NY Med J* 84:832–835, 1906.

440. Sanitary Conditions in Alaska, Including a Report by H. E. Hasseltine, *Public Health Rep* 26:631–636, 1911.

441. Krulish, E.: Sanitary Conditions in Alaska, *Public Health Rep* 28:544, 1913.

442. Murphy, J.A.: The Work of the United States Indian Medical Service, *Survey* 33:444–447, 1914–1915.

443. Rice, P.F.: The Indian Medical Service, *J Lancet* ns 35:429–435, 1915.

444. Eastman, C.A.: The Indians' Health Problem, *Amer Indian Magazine* 4:141, 1916.

445. Newton, E.E.: A Health Campaign Among the Blackfeet Indians, *Rep Lake Mohonk Conf*, Lake Mohonk, NY, 1916, pp 107–111.

446. Middleton, A.E.: Hospitals for Indians Supplanting the Medicine Man, *Mod Hosp* 19:41–44 (July) 1922.

447. Tobey, J.A.: Federal Health Work Among Indians; Account of Health Section of Bureau of Indian Affairs, *Nation's Health* 4:687–689, 1922.

448. Work, H.: Indian Medical Service, *Milit Surg* 55:425–428, 1924.

449. Chesley, A.J.: Is the Indian Susceptible to Health Education? *Amer J Public Health* 15:133–136, 1925.

450. Boynton, R.E., and Hilbert, H.: Government Medical Care Betters Health Conditions of Chippewa Indian Tribes, *Nation's Health* 8:306–366, 1926.

451. Rosebud Reveals the Responsiveness of the Indians; A Health Experience That Won Permanence, *Red Cross Courier* 6:16, 1927.

452. Hoffman, F.L.: Medical and Hospital Service of US Bureau of Indian Affairs, *Hosp Soc Serv* 19:544–552, 1929.

453. Salsbury, C.G.: Medical Work in Navajoland, *Amer J Nurs* 32:415–416, 1932.

454. Indian Service Nurses, *Rep Wisconsin Board of Health* 35:95–98, 1933–1934.

455. Collier, J.: Indian Health Administration, *Proc Conf State Prov Health Author N Amer* 49:40–42, 1934.

456. Sloan, R.P.: White Medicine Man Becomes Indians' Friend (New Phoenix Indian School Hosp.), *Mod Hosp* 43:41–44, 1934.

457. Stone, E.L.: Canadian Indian Medical Services, *Canad Med Ass J* 33:82–85, 1935.

458. Butler, J.J.: Indian Service, *Med Econ* 13:38–46, 1935–1936.

459. Mountin, J.W., and Townsend, J.G.: *Observations on Indian Health Problems and Facilities*, US Dept of Interior, Bull 223, 1936, p 47.

460. Price, W.A.: Eskimo and Indian Field Studies in Alaska and Canada, *J Amer Dent Ass* 23:417–437, 1936.

461. Townsend, J.G.: Health Problems and Federal Health Facilities in the United States, *Proc Conf State Prov Health Author N Amer* 51:93–102, 1936.

462. Townsend, J.G.: *A Statement Relative to the Past, Present, and Future Medical Facilities Provided the Indians in the United States* (attachment to memorandum to Commissioner of Indian Affairs John Collier) (Sept 23) 1936.

463. New General Hospital for Care of Indians, *JAMA* 109:1048, 1937.

464. Watson, E.L.: Indian Hospital, *Hygeia* 17:1110–1113, 1939.

465. Worley, J.F.: Indian Service Health Activities in Alaska, *Health Officer* 4:192–201, 1939.

466. Gerken, E.A.: Development of a Health Education Program, *Amer J Public Health* 30:915–920 (Aug) 1940.

467. Gerken, E.A.: Influencing Health Practices of Primitive People, *Med Wom J* 47:25–30, 1940.

468. Mundt, R.: Indian Medical Service, *Milit Surg* 86:103–106, 1940.

469. Crain, K.C.: US Hospitals Bringing Health to the Native Indians, Eskimos; Government Institutions Surmount Hardship to Achieve Great Work, *Hosp Manage* 53:18 (April) 1942.

470. Hayes, M.: Some Problems of Health in Alaska, *Proc Pacif Sci Conf (6th)* 5:465–472, 1942.

471. McGibony, J.R.: Indians and Selective Service, *Public Health Rep* 57:1–7, 1942.

472. Schnur, L.: Navajos Train Ward Aids to Counteract Medicine Men, *Mod Hosp* 59:80, 1942.

473. Tiber, B.M.: The Indian Service in Alaska, *Amer J Nurs* 42:1114–1118, 1942.

474. McGibony, J.R.: Health Center for 6,000; White Man's Medicine Puts "Indian Sign" on Disease at New Hospital of Pima Agency, *Mod Hosp* 60:60–61, 1943.

475. Radbill, S.X.: Child Hygiene: Chapter in Early American Pediatrics, *Texas Rep Biol Med* 3:419–512, 1945.

476. Moore, P.E.: Indian Health Services, *Canad J Public Health* 37:140–142 (April) 1946.

477. Watson, E.L.: Giving Health Back to the Indians, *Hygeia* 24:750, 1946.

478. Rose, T.H.: Alaska's Hospital Needs, *Alaska's Health* 5:1–7, 1947.

479. Bailey, F.L.: Suggested Techniques for Inducing Navajo Women to Accept Hospitalization During Childbirth and for Implementing Health Education, *Amer J Public Health* 38:1418–1423 (Oct) 1948.

480. Hardenberg, W.: Arctic Sanitation, *Amer J Public Health* 39:202–204 (Feb) 1949.

481. Indian Massacre—New Style, editorial, *Amer J Public Health* 39:1469 (Nov) 1949.

482. Pijoan, M., and McCammon, C.S.: Problem of Medical Care for the Navajo Indians, *JAMA* 140:1013–1015 (July) 1949.

483. Tiber, B.M.: Nursing Among the Navajo Indians, *Amer J Nurs* 49:552–553 (Sept) 1949.

484. Albrecht, C.E.: Health Services and Problems in Alaska, *Amer Public Health Ass Western Branch Ann*, 1950, pp 26–30.

485. *First Five Years of the Alaska Board of Health, A Report to the People of Alaska,* Alaska Dept of Health, 1950, p 26.

486. Foard, F.T.: The Federal Government and American Indians' Health, *JAMA* 142:328–331 (Feb) 1950.

487. Foard, F.T.: Health Services for North American Indians, *Med Wom J* 57:9–16 (Nov) 1950.

488. Twinn, C.R.: Studies on the Biology and Control of Biting Flies in Northern Canada, *Arctic* 2:14–26, 1950.

489. Day, E.K.: Public Health Problems in Alaska: Sewage and Waste Disposal Problems, *Public Health Rep* 66:922–928 (July) 1951.

490. Haldeman, J.C.: Problems of Alaskan Eskimos, Indians, Aleuts, *Public Health Rep* 66:912–917 (July) 1951.

491. Public Health Problems in Alaska, editorial, *Public Health Rep* 66:911 (July) 1951.

492. Review of First Six Years Aboard M.S. Hygiene, Health Department's Pioneer "Floating Health Center," *Alaska's Health* 9:6–7 (Oct) 1951.

493. Wilson, C.S.: Public Health Problems in Alaska: Control of Alaskan Biting Insects, *Public Health Rep* 66:917–922 (July) 1951.

494. Albrecht, C.E.: Public Health in Alaska—United States Frontier, *Amer J Public Health* 42:694–698 (June) 1952.

495. Day, E.K.: Environmental Sanitation Problems in Alaska and Their Solutions, *Harvard Public Health Alumni Bull* 9:3, 1952.

496. DeLien, H., and Hadley, J.N.: How to Recognize an Indian Health Problem, *Hum Org* 11 (No. 3):29–33, 1952.

497. Medical Team Braves Weather to Conduct 30 Clinics for Crippled Children in Interior, *Alaska's Health* 9:3–7 (April) 1952.

498. Young, H.A.: Care of Indians, Eskimos, *Canad Week Bull* 8:5–6 (Dec 12) 1952.

499. Davis, B.M.: Health Program of the Bureau of Indian Affairs, *Milit Surg* 112:171–174, 1953.

500. Old, H.N.: Sanitation Problems of the American Indians, *Amer J Public Health* 43:210–215 (Feb) 1953.

501. Pauls, F.P.: Science and Public Health Research in Alaska, the New Frontier—Enteric Diseases, *Public Health Rep* 68:531–533 (May) 1953.

502. Science and Public Health Research in Alaska, *Public Health Rep* 68:527 (May) 1953.

503. Taylor, M.S.; Van Sandt, M.; and Terry, E.: Consultation by the "Team Method"—Experiment in Bureau of Indian Affairs Hospitals, *Milit Surg* 113:291–294, 1953.

504. Wilson, C.S.: Science and Public Health Research in Alaska, the New Frontier—Mosquito Control, *Public Health Rep* 68:536–537 (May) 1953.

505. Health Survey Team Has Recommendations, *Alaska's Health* 11:1 (Oct) 1954.

506. The Indians' Health and Public Health, editorial, *Amer J Public Health* 44:1461–1462 (Nov) 1954.

507. Moore, P.E.: Health for Indians and Eskimos, *Canad Geogr J* 48:216–221, 1954.

508. Morley, L.A.: Proposed Plan for Selection and Training of Native "Sanitation Aides," *Alaska's Health* 11:3–4 (April) 1954.

509. New Northern Health Service, *Canad Week Bull* 9:5 (May 28) 1954.

510. Parran, T., et al: *Alaska's Health* (summary rep to the US Dept of Interior), U of Pittsburgh Graduate Sch of Public Health, Pittsburgh, Pa, 1954.

511. Sanitation Aide Work Begins for Villages in 3-Way Sponsorship, *Alaska's Health* 11:1–2 (Dec) 1954.

512. French, F.S.; Shaw, J.R.; and Dean, J.D.: The Navajo Health Problem: Its Genesis, Proportions, and a Plan for Its Solution, *Milit Med* 116:451–454, 1955.

513. Haas, L.E., and Simmons, J.J.: What Does the Changing Picture in Public Health Mean to Public Health Education in Personnel Recruitment and Training? Program Design for Meeting Needs, *Amer J Public Health* 46:427–435 (April) 1956.

514. Moore, P.E.: Medical Care of Canada's Indians and Eskimos, *Canad J Public Health* 47:227–233 (June) 1956.

515. Alter, A.J.: Health and Sanitation Problems in the Arctic, *18th Biol Colloq*, 1957, pp 110–118.

516. *Health Services for American Indians*, US Public Health Serv, Div of Indian Health, 1957.

517. Perrott, G. St. J., and West, M.D.: Health Services for American Indians, *Public Health Rep* 72:565–570 (July) 1957.

518. Shaw, J.R.: Guarding the Health of Our Indian Citizens, *Hospitals* 31:38–44 (April 16) 1957.

519. Adair, J., and Deuschle, K.W.: Some Problems of the Physicians on the Navajo Reservation, *Hum Org* 19:19–23, 1958.

520. Aleutian and Northern Villages Included in Sanitation Program, *Alaska's Health* 15:1 (Aug) 1958.

521. The Case of Mary Grey-Eyes, editorial, *Time* (Nov 10) 1958.

522. *Facts About Indian Health*, US Public Health Serv, Div of Indian Health, 1958.

523. *Plan for Medical Facilities Needed for Indian Health Services*, US Public Health Serv, Div of Indian Health, 1958.

524. Zeis, D.M., and Foster, E.: Public Health Nursing in the Forty-ninth State, *Amer J Nurs* 58:1376–1379 (Oct) 1958.

525. Britton, W.B.: The Impact of Hospital Insurance on Indian Health Services, *Med Serv J Canada* 15:632–634 (Nov) 1959.

526. Flemming, A.S.: Indian Health, *Public Health Rep* 74:521–522 (June) 1959.

527. Hildes, J.A.: Medical Problems in the Arctic, *Manitoba Med Rev* 39:581–583, 1959.

528. Jackson, H.C.: Work on EENT Project Continues in Seven Villages in McGrath Area, *Alaska's Health* 16:1–3 (Aug) 1959.

529. Medical School: Indian Fashion, *Wisconsin Med J* 58:668 (Nov) 1959.

530. Parker, L.: Sanitation Aide Villages Stage Clean-Ups, *Alaska's Health* 16:4 (Oct) 1959.

531. Pediatric Evaluations of Indian Children, *Public Health Rep* 74:249–250 (March) 1959.

532. Public Health Nursing for Montana Indians, *Public Health Rep* 74:325–327 (April) 1959.

533. Raup, M.: *The Indian Health Program for 1800–1955*, US

Public Health Serv, Health Serv and Mental Health Administration, Indian Health Serv (March 11) 1959.

534. Willis, J.S.: Northern Health: Problems and Progress, *Northern Affairs Bull* 6:21–25, 1959.

535. Deuschle, K.W., and Adair, J.: An Interdisciplinary Approach to Public Health on the Navajo Indian Reservation: Medical and Anthropological Aspects, *Ann NY Acad Sci* 84:887–905 (Dec) 1960.

536. Hildes, J.A.: Health Problems in the Arctic, *Canad Med Ass J* 83:1255–1257 (Dec) 1960.

537. *Hospital Care in Canada, Recent Trends and Developments,* Dept of Natl Health and Welfare, Res and Statis Div, Ottawa, 1960, p 102.

538. McDermott, W., et al: Introducing Modern Medicine in a Navajo Community, Part I, *Science* 131:197–205 (Jan 22) 1960; Part II, *Science* 131:280–287 (Jan 29) 1960.

539. Simmet, R.: Alaska, Frontier for Health Services, *Public Health Rep* 75:877–912, 1960.

540. Wellman, K.F.: Aktuelle Probleme der öffentlichen Gesundheitspflege bei den Indianern Nordamerikas, *Deutsch Med Wschr* 85:199–209 (Jan 29) 1960.

541. *Sanitation Facilities for Indians,* US Public Health Serv, Health Serv and Mental Health Administration, Indian Health Serv, Publ 735, 1960–1961.

542. Bahl, I.E.: I Couldn't Have Gotten Along Without Sam, *Nurs Outlook* (June) 1961.

543. Casey, J.C.: Progress in Nursing Among Indians in Oklahoma, *Oklahoma J Public Health* 4:6–8, 1961.

544. Hospitals in the Arctic, *Moccasin Telegraph* 21:2, 1961.

545. Hudgins, H.A.: Indian Health Area Led by Oklahoma, *Oklahoma J Public Health* 4:3–5, 1961.

546. Perez, L.K., Jr.: PHS and Indians Join Forces Under Sanitation Facilities Construction Act, *Oklahoma J Public Health* 4:9–11, 1961.

547. Silcott, M.E.: Social Service in Indian Health's Medical Setting, *Oklahoma J Public Health* 4:17–19, 1961.

548. Stevenson, A.H.: Sanitary Facilities Construction Program for

Indians and Alaska Natives, *Public Health Rep* 76:317–322 (April) 1961.

549. Tiber, B.M.: Learning a Brighter Tomorrow, *Oklahoma J Public Health* 4:12–14, 1961.

550. Vincentia, S.: Our Students Learn from the Indians, *Nurs Outlook* 9:356–358 (June) 1961.

551. Wiens, A.A.: Nursing Service on a Chippewa Reservation, *Amer J Nurs* 61:92–93 (April) 1961.

552. Colyar, A.B.: Conference on Medical and Public Health in the Arctic and Antarctic, *Alaska Med* 4:83–84, 1962.

553. Colyar, A.B.: "Some Problems of Disease Prevention and Control in Subarctic and Arctic Areas," Doc 27 in *Conf on Med and Public Health in the Arctic and Antarctic*, WHO, Geneva, 1962, pp 19–25.

554. Griffin, W.: Sanitation Aide Services Are Expanded, *Alaska's Health Welfare* 19:8 (June) 1962.

555. Lantis, M.: *The Alaska Native Village Sanitation Program at the End of Five Years*, US Public Health Serv, Arctic Health Res Center, Anchorage, Alaska, 1962.

556. Mico, P.R.: *Some Implications of the Navajo Health Education Project for Indian Education* (prepared for the 3rd Ann Conf of the Ariz Coordinating Council for Res in Indian Education, Phoenix, Ariz, April 12–13, 1962).

557. Mico, P.R.: A Task for American School Health Education, *J Sch Health* 32:316–320 (Oct) 1962.

558. Patrie, L.E.: A Multiphasic Screening Project on the Pine Ridge Indian Reservation, *J Lancet* 82:511–514 (Dec) 1962.

559. Sanitation Aides to School, *Alaska's Health Welfare* 19:4 (Aug) 1962.

560. Statistics Study Shows Alaska High Death Rates Preventable, *Alaska's Health Welfare* 19:1 (Oct) 1962.

561. Thomas, G.W.: Air Ambulance Service in Northern Newfoundland and Labrador, *Canad Geogr J* 44:16–19, 1962.

562. Wauneka, A.D.: Helping a People to Understand, *Amer J Nurs* 62:88–90 (July) 1962.

563. Whiteford, L.J.: In Service Education: Its Application in the Health Service for Eskimos and Indians, *Canad Nurs* 58:427–429 (May) 1962.

564. Wicks, E.O.: Preventable Disease Deaths Remain Too High, *Alaska's Health Welfare* 19:4–5 (Dec) 1962.

565. Zillatus, M.G.: Public Health Nursing in Papagoland, *Nurs Outlook* 10:792–794 (Dec) 1962.

566. Babbott, F.L., Jr.: "Aspects of Arctic Epidemiology," in *Influence of Cold on Host-Parasite Interactions*, US Arctic Aeromedical Lab, Ft. Wainwright, Alaska, 1963, pp 25–46.

567. Colyar, A.B.: "Some Problems of Disease Prevention and Control in Subarctic and Arctic Areas," Publ 18 in *Conf on Med and Public Health in the Arctic and Antarctic*, WHO, Geneva, 1963.

568. Conference on Medicine and Public Health in the Arctic and Antarctic, *WHO Techn Rep Ser*, No. 253, 1963, p 27.

569. Deuschle, K.W.: Training and Use of Medical Auxiliaries in a Navajo Community, *Public Health Rep* 78:461–469 (June) 1963.

570. Loughlin, B.W.: Aide Training Reaches the Navajo Reservation, *Amer J Nurs* 63:106–109 (July) 1963.

571. *Medicine and Public Health in the Arctic and Antarctic— Selected Papers from a Conference*, WHO, Geneva, 1963, p 169.

572. Peters, J.P.: Health Services to the American Indian, *Westerner's New York Posse Brand Book* 10 (No. 3):1–6, 1963.

573. Roberts, B.J.; Mico, P.R.; and Clark, W.: An Experimental Study of Two Approaches to Communication, *Amer J Public Health* 53:1361–1381 (Sept) 1963.

574. Seltzer, R.A.: Multiphasic Screening Project in an Indian School, *Public Health Rep* 78:971–976 (Nov) 1963.

575. *Trends in Indian Health and Health Services, 1961 and 1962*, US Public Health Serv, Div of Indian Health, 1963.

576. Whiteford, L.J.: Nursing with INHS in the Saskatchewan Region, *Canad Nurs* 59:365–368 (April) 1963.

577. AMA Helping Indians, *AMA News*, March 2, 1964.

578. Findley, D.: Some Health Problems of the Navajo Indians, *Nebraska State Med J* 49:326–332, 1964.

579. *Health of Florida's Indians*, Jacksonville, Fla: Fla State Board of Health, 1964.

580. Hickey, J.L.S.: Electric Power and Environmental Health

in Alaska Native Villages, *Public Health Rep* 79:1087–1092 (June) 1964.

581. Lees, B.: Government Controlled Medicine—Facts and Figures, *Clin Med* 71:1323–1326 (Aug) 1964.

582. Wagner, C.J.: Federal Health Services for Indians and Alaskan Natives, *J Lancet* 84:289 (Sept) 1964.

583. Wagner, C.J., and Rabeau, E.S.: Indian Poverty and Indian Health, *Health, Education, and Welfare Indicators* (March) 1964, pp xxiv–xlix.

584. Wilson, M.R.: Effect of the Alaska Earthquake on Functions of PHS Hospital, *Public Health Rep* 79:853–862 (Oct) 1964.

585. Woodville, L.: Healthier Indian Mothers and Babies, *Public Health Rep* 79:468 (June) 1964.

586. *Sanitation Facilities for Indians*, US Public Health Serv, Div of Indian Health, Publ 735, 1964–1967.

587. For Healthier Little Indians, *Today's Health* 43:12 (July) 1965.

588. Nowak, J.: Radiologist Serves 50,000 Indians, *Your Radiologist* 8 (Fall) 1965.

589. Nurses in the North, *Canada's Health Welfare* 20:2–3 (Jan 8) 1965.

590. Rath, O.J.S.: Public Health Practice Among the Indian Population, *Manitoba Med Rev* 45:644–646, 1965.

591. Thompson, S., and Tyler, I.: Cultural Factors in Casework Treatment with Long-term Hospitalization of Navajo Patients, *Soc Casework J* (April) 1965, p 1.

592. Carlile, W.K.: Division of Indian Health Pediatric Residency Program, abstracted, *Proc 1st Joint Meeting of the Clin Soc and Commissioned Officers Ass USPHS*, Baltimore, Md (May) 1966, p 10.

593. Gallina, J.N.: Unit-Dose Dispensing of Injectables at a PHS Indian Health Center, abstracted, *Proc 1st Joint Meet of the Clin Soc and Commissioned Officers Ass USPHS*, Baltimore, Md (May) 1966, p 37.

594. *The Indian Health Program of the US*, rev ed, US Public Health Serv, Div of Indian Health, Publ 1026, 1966.

595. Indian Village in the Grand Canyon, *Nurs Outlook* 14:1 (March) 1966.

596. Jonz, W.W.: Staffing Health Education Programs for American Indians, *Public Health Rep* 81:627–630 (July) 1966.

597. Knight, J.L.: Refilling Outpatient Prescriptions at a PHS Indian Hospital, abstracted, *Proc 2nd Joint Meet of the Clin Soc and Commissioned Officers Ass USPHS*, Baltimore, Md (May) 1966, p 13.

598. Martens, E.G.: Culture and Communications—Training Indians and Eskimos as Community Health Workers, *Canad J Public Health* 57:495–503 (Nov) 1966.

599. *Operation SAM—Applied Research in Health Program Management* (Proc 1st Orientation Conf, Nov 14, 1966), US Public Health Serv, Div of Indian Health, 1966.

600. Something New in Training Indian and Eskimo Health Workers, *Canad J Public Health* 57:535 (Nov) 1966.

601. Stevenson, A.H., and Johnson, C.C.: Designing an Environmental Health Activity for an Underprivileged People, abstracted, *Proc 1st Joint Meet of the Clin Soc and Commissioned Officers Ass USPHS*, Baltimore, Md (May) 1966, p 9.

602. Sumpter, G.: White "Medicine Man," *New Physician* 15: A–10, 11, 86, 87 (May) 1966.

603. Baizerman, M.: The Community Organization Method of Social Work in a Public Health Service Hospital, abstracted, *Proc 2nd Joint Meet of the Clin Soc and Commissioned Officers Ass USPHS*, Atlanta, Ga (May) 1967, p 55.

604. Bock, G.E.: The Medicine Men, *PHS World* 2:32–34 (April) 1967.

605. Casselman, E.: Public Health Nursing Services for Indians, *Canad J Public Health* 58:543–546 (Dec) 1967.

606. *HPSC Current Project Summaries and Published Monograph Abstracts—1967* (Operation SAM for the development of a comprehensive Indian Health Program, Tucson, Arizona), US Public Health Serv, Div of Indian Health, Health Program Systems Center, Tucson, Ariz, 1967.

607. Indian, Alaskan Health Below Par but Improving, *Med Tribune* 8:24B (March 4) 1967.

608. Murray, W.W.: The Satellite Physical Therapy Clinic Within

the Window Rock Field Office Area, abstracted, *Proc 2nd Joint Meet of the Clin Soc and Commissioned Officers Ass USPHS,* Atlanta, Ga (May) 1967, p 67.

609. *Operation SAM—A Systems Analysis Module for the Development of a Comprehensive Indian Health Program: Evaluation of a Trial Source—Data Collection System,* US Public Health Serv, Div of Indian Health, Health Program Systems Center, Tucson, Ariz (June) 1967.

610. *Sanitation Facilities for Indians—What Does P.L. 86–121 Mean to You,* US Public Health Serv, Div of Indian Health, 1967.

611. Steinmetz, N.: Pediatric Services and Residency Training in the Canadian Arctic, *Canad J Public Health* 58:461–463 (Oct) 1967.

612. Towsley, A.C.: The Doctor's Wife: Assignment: Indian Reservation, *Med World News,* May 19, 1967.

613. Anderson, M.W.: *Social Work in Maternal and Child Health Programs,* Berkeley: U of Calif Press, 1968.

614. Deacon, W.E.: Evaluation of the Community Health Aid Program, Pine Ridge, South Dakota, abstracted, *Proc 3rd Joint Meet of the Clin Soc and Commissioned Officers Ass USPHS,* San Francisco, Calif (March) 1968, p 73.

615. Freestone, A.: Environmental Sanitation in Indian Reserves, *Canad J Public Health* 59:25–27 (Jan) 1968.

616. *Health Concepts and Attitudes of the Papago Indians,* US Public Health Serv, Div of Indian Health, Health Program Systems Center, Tucson, Ariz (Sept) 1968.

617. *Health Program Evaluation: Impact Study of the Indian Sanitation Facilities Construction Act,* US Public Health Serv, Div of Indian Health, Health Program Systems Center, Tucson, Ariz, 1968.

618. *The Indian Health Program of the US Public Health Service,* rev ed, US Public Health Serv, Div of Indian Health, Publ 1394, 1968.

619. *Indian Health Service Newsletter,* US Public Health Serv, Health Serv and Mental Health Administration, Indian Health Serv 1 (No. 1) (Dec) 1968.

620. Knight, J.L.: Simplified Nursing Station Narcotic-Hypnotic

System with Automatic Stock Replenishment, abstracted, *Proc 3rd Joint Meet of the Clin Soc and Commissioned Officers Ass USPHS*, San Francisco, Calif (March) 1968, p 17.

621. Lo, The Poor Indian, editorial, *New Eng J Med* 278:47–48 (Jan 4) 1968.

622. *Premise and Home—Environmental Health Survey*, US Public Health Serv, Indian Health Serv, Health Program Systems Center, Tucson, Ariz, 1968.

623. Procter, H.A.: The Husbandry of a Northern Health Service, *Arch Environ Health* 17:462–463 (Nov) 1968.

624. Steinmetz, N.: Pediatric Needs in the Arctic, a Challenge and an Opportunity, *Clin Pediat* 7:498–504 (Aug) 1968.

625. They Matched the Mountains, *Public Health Serv World* (March) 1968, p 1.

626. USPHS Regulations, or, "Once a Beneficiary, Always a Beneficiary . . . ," *Alaska Med* 10:187–189, 1968.

627. Varied Health Needs Met at Indian Schools, *Public Health Serv World* (Sept–Oct) 1968, pp 27–28.

628. *Your Government and the Indian*, US Public Health Serv, Div of Indian Health, 1968.

629. Bowman, C.R.: The Environmental Health Program of the Alaska Area Native Health Service, *Alaska Med* 11:128–129, 1969.

630. Coulter, P.O., et al: Parallel Experience: An Interview Technique, *Amer J Nurs* 69:1028–1030 (May) 1969.

631. DeMontigny, L.H., and Parks, G.: The Muckleshoot Indians Use of Multi-Disciplined Resources in Effecting a Comprehensive Health Program, abstracted, *Proc 4th Joint Meet of the Clin Soc and Commissioned Officers Ass USPHS*, Boston (June) 1969, p 64.

632. Gilbert, R.: Do Indian Patients Use Their Medication? abstracted, *Proc 4th Joint Meet of the Clin Soc and Commissioned Officers Ass USPHS*, Boston (June) 1969, p 73.

633. *The Indian Health Program of the US Public Health Service, 1955–1969*, US Public Health Serv, Health Serv and Mental Health Administration, Indian Health Serv, Publ 1394, 1969.

634. *The Indian Health Program of the US Public Health Service,*

1955–1969, rev ed, US Public Health Serv, Health Serv and Mental Health Administration, Indian Health Serv, Publ 1026, 1969.

635. *Indian Health Service Newsletter*, US Public Health Serv, Health Serv and Mental Health Administration, Indian Health Serv 1 (No. 2) (March) 1969.

636. *Indian Health Service Newsletter*, US Public Health Serv, Health Serv and Mental Health Administration, Indian Health Serv 1 (No. 3) (June) 1969.

637. Lee, J.F.: Response to the December Issue 1968 of "Alaska Medicine," letter to the editor, *Alaska Med* 11:3–6, 1969.

638. Michael, J.M.: Experience of the Public Health Service in Training and Using Health Auxiliaries, *Public Health Rep* 84:681–689 (Aug) 1969.

639. Nowak, J.: What's Happening with the Indians? *HSMHA World* 4:29–32 (Sept–Oct) 1969.

640. Portney, G.L.: A Computerized Projected Analysis of the Indian Health Service Family Planning Program, abstracted, *Proc 4th Joint Meet of the Clin Soc and Commissioned Officers Ass USPHS*, Boston (June) 1969, p 76.

641. *The Professional Sanitarian in the Indian Health Service*, US Public Health Serv, Health Serv and Mental Health Administration, Indian Health Serv, 1969.

642. Rabeau, E.S., and Reaud, A.: Evaluation of PHS Program Providing Family Planning Services for American Indians, *Amer J Public Health* 59:1331–1338 (Aug) 1969.

643. Rubensten, A., et al: Effect of Improved Sanitary Facilities on Infant Diarrhea in a Hopi Village, *Public Health Rep* 85: 1093–1097 (Dec) 1969.

644. Rymer, S.: New Approaches to Health Problems of the Indian and Eskimo People, *Canad Med Ass J* 101:93–94 (Nov 15) 1969.

645. Schlafman, I.H.: Health Systems Research to Deliver Comprehensive Services to Indians, *Public Health Rep* 84:697–704 (Aug) 1969.

646. Shook, D.C.: Alaska Native Community Health Aide Training, *Alaska Med* 11:1–5, 1969.

647. Uhrich, R.B.: Tribal Community Health Representatives of

the Indian Health Service, *Public Health Rep* 84:965–970
(Nov) 1969.

V. INFECTIOUS AGENTS AND DISEASES

A. GENERAL AND UNSPECIFIED

648. *(Fourth) Annual Report of Bureau of American Ethnology,
1882–1883,* Smithsonian Inst, Bur of Amer Ethnology, 1886,
pp 108, 136, 146.

649. Webb, D.W.: The Indian Under Medical Observation, *Proc
Florida Med Ass,* 1887, pp 27–34.

650. Syphilis and Tuberculosis Among the American Indian, *Med
Analectic* (Nov 1) 1888.

651. *(Fourteenth) Annual Report of the Bureau of American
Ethnology, 1892–1893,* Smithsonian Inst, Bur of Amer Ethnology, 1896, p 830.

652. *(Twenty-sixth) Annual Report of the Bureau of American
Ethnology, 1904–1905,* Smithsonian Inst, Bur of Amer Ethnology, 1908, pp 52, 53, 55, 58, 64, 156, 185, 267.

653. Thomas, R.E.: The Influence of Mixed Blood upon the Susceptibility to Infection in the American Indian, *Southern
Calif Practitioner* 25:576, 1910.

654. *Contagious and Infectious Diseases Among the Indians*
(letter from the Secretary of the Treasury), 62nd Congress,
3rd Session, US Senate, Doc 1038, 1913, p 85.

655. Price, W.A.: Some Causes for Change in Susceptibility of
Eskimos and Indians to Acute and Chronic Infections upon
Contact with Modern Civilization, *J Dent Res* 14:230–231,
1934.

656. Marchand, J.F.: Tribal Epidemics in the Yukon, *JAMA* 123:
1019–1020 (Dec) 1943.

657. Honigmann, J.J.: Tribal Epidemics in the Yukon, Comment,
JAMA 124:386 (Feb) 1944.

658. Greenberg, L.; Blake, J.D.; and Connel, M.F.: An Immu-

nological Study of the Canadian Indian, *Canad Med Ass J* 77:211–216 (Aug) 1957.

659. Maddy, K.T., et al: *Coccidioidin, Histoplasmin, and Tuberculin Sensitivity of Students in Selected High Schools and Colleges in Arizona*, US Public Health Serv, Publ 575, 1957, pp 121–126.

660. Mills, L.F.: Epidemic in a Navajo School, *Bull Menninger Clin* 26:189–194 (July) 1962.

660A. Lindert, M.C.; Pandola, G.; and Taugher, P.J.: CPC: Whipple's Disease in an American Indian, *Marquette Med Rev* 30:79–84, 1964.

661. Albrecht, C.E.: Eradication of Some Arctic Infectious Diseases, *Arch Environ Health* 17:668–675 (Oct) 1968.

B. PARTIALLY SPECIFIED

i. Upper and Lower Respiratory Infections

662. *Eye, Ear, Nose, and Throat Infections in Alaska*, Alaska Dept of Health, 1956.

663. Hayman, C.R., and Kester, F.E.: Eye, Ear, Nose, and Throat Infection in Natives of Alaska, *Northwest Med* 56:423–430 (April) 1957.

664. *The McGrath Project, Documentation on Study and Prevention of Upper Respiratory Diseases*, US Public Health Serv, Arctic Health Res Center, Anchorage, Alaska, 1962.

665. Justice, J.W.: Respiratory Disease Epidemic in Hoonah, Southeast Alaska, *Alaska Med* 7:30–34, 1965.

666. Mandell, G.L., and Prosnitz, L.R.: Peritonsillar Abscess and Cellulitis, *New York J Med* 66:2667–2669 (Oct) 1966.

667. Proceedings of the Fourth National Conference on Indian Health, I: Respiratory Infections, *Arch Environ Health* 17: 247–266 (Aug) 1968.

668. Upadhyay, Y.N., and Gerrard, J.W.: Recurrent Pneumonia in Indian Children, *Ann Allerg* 27:218–224 (May) 1969.

ii. Gastrointestinal Infections

669. (*Third*) *Annual Report of the Bureau of American Eth-*

nology, 1881–1882, Smithsonian Inst, Bur of Amer Ethnology, 1884, p 265.

670. Spector, B.K., and Hardy, A.V.: Studies of the Acute Diarrheal Diseases, II: Parasitological Observations, *Public Health Rep* 54:1105–1113 (June) 1939.

671. Frank, I.: Treatment of Epidemic Diarrheas on the Reservation, *Arizona Med* 6:35–36, 1949.

672. Gitlitz, I.: Diarrheal Diseases on an Indian Reservation, *Arizona Med* 7:42–44, 1950 .

673. Pauls, F.P.: Enteric Diseases in Alaska, *Arctic* 6:205–212, 1953.

674. Gordon, J.E.; Babbott, F.L., Jr.; and Babbott, J.G.: *Transmission of Intestinal Pathogens in Polar Climates: Field Studies on Intestinal Infestations in Alaska*, Commission on Environmental Hygiene, US Armed Forces Epidemiological Board, Ann Rep (March 1) 1955–(Feb 28) 1956, p 44.

675. Babbott, J.G.; Babbott, F.L., Jr.; and Gordon, J.E.: Arctic Environment and Intestinal Infection, *Amer J Med Sci* 231:338–360 (May) 1956.

676. Fournelle, F., and Cullinson, S.: Enteric Diseases in Alaska, *Amer J Med Tech* (special issue) 22:36, 1956.

677. Gordon, J.E., and Babbott, F.L., Jr.: Acute Intestinal Infection in Alaska, *Public Health Rep* 74:49–54 (Jan) 1959.

678. Gordon, J.E., and Babbott, F.L., Jr.: Acute Intestinal Infection in the Arctic, *Amer J Public Health* 49:1441–1453 (Nov) 1959.

679. Goodwin, M.H.: Status of Some Infectious Enteric Diseases in Arizona, *Arizona Med* 21:619–627, 1964.

680. Lasersohn, W.: Acute Diarrheal Disease in Zuni Community, *Public Health Rep* 80:457–461 (May) 1965.

681. Fournelle, H.J.; Rader, V.; and Allen, C.: A Survey of Enteric Infections Among Alaskan Indians, *Public Health Rep* 81:797–803 (Sept) 1966.

682. Proceedings of the Fourth National Conference on Indian Health, II: Enteric Infections, *Arch Environ Health* 18:358–378 (March) 1969.

iii. Central Nervous System Infections

683. Seid, S.E.: Meningitis Epidemic Among Navajo Indians, *JAMA* 115:923–924, 1940.

iv. Parasitic Infestations

684. Owen, W.B.; Honess, R.E.; and Simon, J.R.: Protozoal Infestations of Children, *JAMA* 102:913–915, 1934.

685. Parnell, I.N.: Animal Parasites of Northeast Canada, *Canad Field Naturalist* 48:111–130, 1934.

686. Saunders, L.G.: A Survey of Helminth and Protozoan Incidence in Man and Dogs at Fort Chipewyan, Alberta, *J Parasit* 35:31–34 (Feb) 1949.

687. Cameron, T.W.M.: Parasitology and the Arctic, *Trans Royal Soc Canada*, 3rd Ser, 51 (section 5):1–10, 1957.

688. Cameron, T.W.M.: "Parasitological Problems in High Latitudes, with Particular Reference to Canada," Doc 16 in *Conf on Med and Public Health in the Arctic and Antarctic*, WHO, Geneva, 1962, p 9.

689. Melvin, D.M., and Brooke, M.M.: Parasitologic Surveys on Indian Reservations in Montana, South Dakota, New Mexico, Arizona, and Wisconsin, *Amer J Trop Med* 11:765–772 (Nov) 1962.

690. Becker, D.A.: Enteric Parasites of Indians and Anglo-Americans on the Winnebago and Omaha Reservations in Nebraska, *Nebraska State Med J* 53:293–296 (June) 1968.

C. Diseases Transmitted from Man to Man

i. Viral

a. General

691. Van Rooyen, C.E.: Serologic Surveys of Arctic Populations and Some Virus Diseases of Interest, *Arch Environ Health* 17:547–554 (Oct) 1968.

b. Polio

692. Adamson, J.D.: Poliomyelitis in the Arctic, *Canad Med Ass J* 61:339–348 (Oct) 1949.

693. Adamson, J.D.; Bow, M.R.; and Lossing, E.H.: Poliomyelitis in the Yukon, *Canad J Public Health* 45:337–344 (Aug) 1954.

694. MacDonald, R.A.: Poliomyelitis Epidemic on a Minnesota Indian Reservation, *Minnesota Med* 43:842–844 (Dec) 1960.

695. Reinhard, K.R., and Gerloff, R.K.: Immunity Toward Poliovirus Among Alaskan Natives, II: A Serologic Survey of 47 Native Communities of Western and Northern Alaska, *Amer J Hyg* 72:298–307 (Sept) 1960.

696. Reinhard, K.R., and Gibson, H.V.: Immunity Toward Poliovirus Among Alaskan Natives, I: Comparative Reported Incidence of Clinical Poliomyelitis in Alaskan Natives and Non-Native Residents, 1950–54, *Amer J Hyg* 72:289–297 (Sept) 1960.

697. Fieldsteel, A.H., and Chin, T.D.Y.: An Epidemiologic and Immunologic Study of Poliomyelitis on an Indian Reservation, *Amer J Hyg* 76:1–14 (July) 1962.

c. Viral Meningitis

698. Oren, J., et al: Aseptic Meningitis on an Indian Reservation: An Epidemic Associated with ECHO 9 Virus, *Amer J Dis Child* 102:843–852 (Dec) 1961.

d. Influenza

699. Treon, F.: Epidemic Influenza Among the Sioux Indians, *Cincinnati Lancet–Clin* ns 24:160, 1890.

700. Influenza Among American Indians, *Public Health Rep* 34:1008–1009, 1919.

701. Influenza Among the American Indians, *Amer J Phys Anthrop* 3:193–194, 1920.

702. Lackman, D.B., et al: A Comparison of Influenza in the Northwestern United States Caused by A-Prime and Asian Influenza Viruses, *Canad J Public Health* 50:71–79 (Feb) 1959.

703. Maynard, J.E.: Influenza B at Fort Yukon: Report of an Outbreak, 1961, *Alaska Med* 4:1–6, 1962.

704. Philip, R.N., and Lackman, D.B.: Observations on the Present Distributions of Influenza A Swine Antibodies Among Alaskan Natives Relative to the Occurrence of Influenza in 1913–1919, *Amer J Hyg* 75:322–334 (May) 1962.

705. Dobson, P.M., et al: Epidemic Virus Influenza in Nova Scotia and New Brunswick During the First Six Months in 1963, *Med Serv J Canada* 19:799–808, 1963.

e. Respiratory Viral Infections

706. Hildes, J.A., et al: Surveys of Respiratory Virus Antibodies in an Arctic Indian Population, *Canad Med Ass J* 93:1015–1018 (Nov) 1965.

707. Gard, S.: Respiratory Virus Infections Other than Influenza, *Arch Environ Health* 17:543–546 (Oct) 1968.

f. Hepatitis

708. Davis, T.R.A.: Infectious Hepatitis in Two Arctic Villages, abstracted, *Sci in Alaska*, Proc 7th Alaskan Sci Conf (1956), AAAS, Alaska Div, p 94.

709. Davis, T.R.A.: *An Outbreak of Infectious Hepatitis in Two Arctic Villages*, US Arctic Aeromedical Lab, Ladd Air Force Base, Alaska, Techn Note 56–38, 1956, p 14.

710. Aach, D., et al: Efficacy of Varied Doses of Gamma Globulin During an Epidemic of Infectious Hepatitis, Hoonah, Alaska, 1961, *Amer J Public Health* 53:1623–1629 (Oct) 1963.

711. Maynard, J.E.: Infectious Hepatitis at Fort Yukon, Alaska—Report of an Outbreak, 1960–1961, *Amer J Public Health* 53:31–39 (Jan) 1963.

712. McCollum, R.W.: Hepatitis As It Relates to the Arctic, *Arch Environ Health* 17:529–536 (Oct) 1968.

g. Enteroviruses

713. Reinhard, K.R.: Ecology of Enteroviruses in the Western

American Arctic, *Acta Path Microbiol Scand*, Suppl 154, pp 332–333, 1962.

714. Reinhard, K.R.: Notes on the Ecology of Enteroviruses in Western, Northern and Central Alaska, abstracted, *Sci in Alaska*, Proc 12th Alaskan Sci Conf (1961), AAAS, Alaska Div, 1962, pp 184–185.

715. Reinhard, K.R.: "The Ecology of Enteroviruses in Alaska," in *Influence of Cold on Host-Parasite Interactions*, US Arctic Aeromedical Lab, Ft. Wainwright, Alaska, 1963, pp 47–88.

716. Reinhard, K.R.: Ecology of Enteroviruses in the Western Arctic, *JAMA* 183:410–418 (Feb) 1963.

h. Smallpox

717. Schoolcraft, H.R.: *Information Respecting the History, Condition, and Prospects of the Indian Tribes of the United States*, vol 1, Philadelphia: Lippincott, Grambo and Co, 1852, p 257.

718. (*Fifteenth*) *Annual Report of the Bureau of American Ethnology, 1893–1894*, Smithsonian Inst, Bur of Amer Ethnology, 1896, pp 191–199.

719. (*Nineteenth*) *Annual Report of the Bureau of American Ethnology, 1897–1898*, Smithsonian Inst, Bur of Amer Ethnology, 1900, pp 36, 61, 171–172.

720. (*Twenty-seventh*) *Annual Report of the Bureau of American Ethnology, 1905–1906*, Smithsonian Inst, Bur of Amer Ethnology, 1911, p 620.

721. Heagerty, J.J.: Smallpox Among Indians of Canada, *Public Health Rep* 17:51–61 (Feb) 1926.

722. (*Forty-fifth*) *Annual Report of the Bureau of American Ethnology, 1927–1928*, Smithsonian Inst, Bur of Amer Ethnology, 1930, pp 212, 315.

723. (*Forty-sixth*) *Annual Report of the Bureau of American Ethnology, 1928–1929*, Smithsonian Inst, Bur of Amer Ethnology, 1930, p 396.

724. Pusey, W.A.: Smallpox Epidemic Among the Mandan Indians in 1837, *JAMA* 95:1992–1994 (Dec) 1930.

725. Stearn, E.A., and Stearn, A.E.: *The Effect of Smallpox on the*

Destiny of the American Indian, Boston: Bruce Humphries, 1945.

726. Duffy, J.: Smallpox and the Indians in the American Colonies, *Bull Hist Med* 25:324–341 (July–Aug) 1951.

i. Measles

727. Peart, A.F.W., and Nagler, F.P.: Measles in the Canadian Arctic, 1952, *Canad J Public Health* 45:146–156 (April) 1954.

728. Foster, S.O.: *Measles Epidemic on the Fort Apache Indian Reservation,* US Public Health Serv, Rep 8 (Sept) 1962.

729. Van Arsdell, W., and Dietz, J.: Measles Among the Navajo, abstracted, *Proc 2nd Joint Meet of the Clin Soc and Commissioned Officers Ass USPHS,* Atlanta, Ga (May) 1967, p 30.

ii. Trachoma

730. Fox, L.W.: Trachoma Problem Among North American Indians, *JAMA* 86:404–406, 1926.

731. Chesley, A.J.: Prevalence of Trachoma Among Indians of Northwest, *Eye Ear Nose Throat Mon* 6:395, 1927.

732. Guthrie, M.C.: Indian Service Part in Control of Trachoma, *Eye Ear Nose Throat Mon* 6:399–401, 1927.

733. Posey, W.C.: Observations of Trachoma Among Indians, *Eye Ear Nose Throat Mon* 6:402, 1927.

734. Posey, W.C.: Trachoma Among Indians of the Southwest, *JAMA* 88:1618–1619, 1927.

735. Crouch, J.H.: A Trachoma Survey of 29 Public Schools on or Near Indian Reservations in Montana, *Public Health Rep* 44:637–645, 1929.

736. Fox, L.W.: The Indian and the Trachoma Problem, *Amer J Ophthal* 12:457–468, 1929.

737. Warner, H.J.: Results of Trachoma Work by the Indian Service in Arizona and New Mexico, *Public Health Rep* 44:2913–2930, 1929.

738. Byers, W.G.M.: Trachoma in Canada, *Canad Med Ass J* 27:372–376, 1932.

739. Wall, J.J.: Trachoma Among Indians of Western Canada, *Canad Public Health J* 25:279–283, 1934.

740. Wall, J.J.: Trachoma in Indians of Western Canada, *Brit J Ophthal* 18:524–532, 1934.

741. Tillim, S.J.: Trachoma Among Indians, *Sightsav Rev* 5:176–186, 1935.

742. Eilers, P.G.: Fifteen Years with Trachoma Among Indians, *Southwest Med* 20:457–460, 1936.

743. Hancock, J.C.: Trachoma Treatment at Fort Apache "Trachoma School," *Southwest Med* 21:80–83, 1937.

744. Thygeson, P.: Trachomatous Keratitis (Pannus); Biomicroscopic Study of 280 Indian School Children, *Arch Ophthal* 17:18–26, 1937.

745. Townsend, J.G.: Trachoma Control in the Indian Service (Use of Sulfanilamide), *Sightsav Rev* 9:280–289, 1939.

746. Julianelle, L.A., and Smith, J.E.: A Statistical Analysis of Clinical Trachoma, *Amer J Ophthal* 26:158–165, 1943.

747. Forster, W.G., and McGibony, J.R.: Trachoma, *Amer J Ophthal* 27:1107–1117, 1944.

748. Siniscal, A.A.: Epidemiological Aspects of Trachoma in USA, *Bull WHO* 16:1047–1050, 1957.

749. Cady, L.D.: Study of *Trachoma dubium, Amer J Ophthal* 45:41–43 (Jan) 1958.

750. Cobb, J.C., and Dawson, C.R.: Trachoma Among the Southwestern Indians, *JAMA* 175:405–406 (Feb) 1961.

751. Hanna, L.: Isolation of Trachoma and Inclusion Conjunctivitis Viruses in the United States, *Ann NY Acad Sci* 98:24–30 (March) 1962.

752. Foster, S.O.: Trachoma in an American Indian Village, *Public Health Rep* 80:829–832 (Aug) 1965.

753. Foster, S.O.; Posers, D.K.; and Thygeson, P.: Trachoma Therapy: A Controlled Study, *Amer J Ophthal* 61:451–455 (March) 1966.

754. Dawson, C.R.: Controlled Treatment Trials of Trachoma in American Indian Children, *Lancet* 2:961 (Nov) 1967.

755. Powers, D.K.; Hoshiwara, I.; and Krutz, G.: Preliminary Report: Comprehensive Trachoma Control Program Among the

Southwest American Indians, abstracted, *Proc 2nd Joint Meet of the Clin Soc and Commissioned Officers Ass USPHS*, Atlanta, Ga (May) 1967, p 49.

756. Hoshiwara, I., and Krutz, G.: Comprehensive Trachoma Survey and Treatment Program Among the Southwest Indians in the Phoenix Area: Results of 18 Months Experience, abstracted, *Proc 3rd Joint Meet of the Clin Soc and Commissioned Officers Ass USPHS*, San Francisco, Calif (March) 1968, p 27.

757. Philip, R.N., et al: An Epidemiologic and Laboratory Study of Trachoma on the Northern Cheyenne Indian Reservation, abstracted, *Proc 3rd Joint Meet of the Clin Soc and Commissioned Officers Ass USPHS*, San Francisco, Calif (March) 1968, p 27.

758. Biswell, R.: Keratoplasty and Trachoma in the Southwestern Indian, *Arch Ophthal* 81:791–796 (June) 1969.

759. Hoshiwara, I., and Krutz, G.: Comprehensive Trachoma Survey Among the Southwestern Indian Tribes: Summary of 30 Months Experience, abstracted, *Proc 4th Joint Meet of the Clin Soc and Commissioned Officers Ass USPHS*, Boston (June) 1969, p 15.

760. Lawler, D.: Trachoma Control Activity on the Navajo Indian Reservation, abstracted, *Proc 4th Joint Meet of the Clin Soc and Commissioned Officers Ass USPHS*, Boston (June) 1969, p 15.

iii. Bacteria (Excluding Tuberculosis)

a. Bacterial Bronchitis and Pneumonias

761. Reinhard, K.R.: Bacteriological Findings in the McGrath, Alaska, Ear, Nose, and Throat Project, abstracted, *Sci in Alaska*, Proc 13th Alaskan Sci Conf (1962), AAAS, Alaska Div, 1963.

762. Herbert, F.A., et al: Pneumonia in Indian and Eskimo Infants and Children, Part I: A Clinical Study, *Canad Med Ass J* 96:257–264 (Feb) 1967.

763. Mahon, W.A., et al: Pneumonia in Indian and Eskimo Infants

and Children, Part II: A Controlled Clinical Trial of Antibiotics, *Canad Med Ass J* 96:265–268 (Feb) 1967.

b. Streptococci Producing Scarlet Fever and Rheumatic Fever

764. Sherwood, N.P.; Nigg, C.; and Baumgartner, L.: Studies on the Dick Test and Natural Immunity to Scarlet Fever Among the American Indians, *J Immun* 11:343–360, 1926.

765. Frank, M.L., and Elkin, C.A.: Scarlet Fever Among Pueblo Indians: Observations on Susceptibility and Occurrence, *Amer J Dis Child* 71:477–481, 1946.

766. Newton, J.K.: Scarlet Fever Among the Pueblo Indians, *Amer J Dis Child* 72:490–491, 1946.

767. Zimmerman, R.A.: A Streptococcal Epidemic in an Isolated Civilian Population with Institution of Mass Prophylaxis, *J Pediat* 69:40–45, 1966.

768. Bennett, P.H.: "Rheumatic Fever in Indians," in Bennett, P.H., and Wood, H.N. (eds.): *Population Studies in Rheumatic Diseases*, New York: Excerpta Med Found, 1968.

c. Nephritogenic Streptococci

769. Kleinman, H.: Epidemic Acute Glomerulonephritis at Red Lake, *Minnesota Med* 37:479–483, 1954.

770. Reinstein, C.R.: Epidemic Nephritis at Red Lake, Minnesota, *J Pediat* 47:25–34 (July) 1955.

771. Updyke, E.L.; Moore, M.S.; and Conroy, E.: Provisional New Type of Group A Streptococci Associated with Nephritis, *Science* 121:171–172 (Feb) 1955.

772. Bone, M.; Braude, F.F.; and Kleinman, H.: Complement-Fixing Antibody Response to M-Protein of Nephritogenic Streptococci in Glomerulonephritis, *J Lab Clin Med* 50:705–711 (Nov) 1957.

773. Perlman, L.V., et al: Poststreptococcal Glomerulonephritis: A Ten-Year Followup of an Epidemic, *JAMA* 194:175–182 (Oct) 1965.

774. Anthony, B.F., et al: Epidemic Acute Nephritis with Reap-

pearance of Type-49 Streptococcus, *Lancet* 2:787–789 (Oct) 1967.

775. Anthony, B.F.; Perlman, L.V.; and Wannamaker, L.W.: Skin Infections and Acute Nephritis in American Indian Children, *Pediatrics* 39:263–279 (Feb) 1967.

776. Maxted, W.R.; Fraser, C.A.M.; and Parker, M.T.: Streptococcus Pyogenes, Type 49: A Nephritogenic Streptococcus with a Wide Geographical Distribution, *Lancet* 1:641–644 (Sept) 1967.

777. Perlman, L.V.; Herdman, R.C.; and Vernier, R.: Post-Streptococcal Glomerulonephritis, a 10-Year Followup of an Epidemic, abstracted, *Proc 3rd Joint Meet of the Clin Soc and Commissioned Officers Ass USPHS*, San Francisco, Calif (March) 1968, p 77.

d. Staphylococci

778. Dillenberg, H., and Waldron, M.P.D.: A Preventive Approach to Impetigo of Treaty Indians Using Staphylococcus Polyvalent Somatic Antigen Vaccine, *Canad Med Ass J* 89:947–949 (Nov) 1963.

779. Anthony, B.F.; Giebink, G.S.; and Quie, P.Q.: Neomycin-Resistant Staphylococci in a Rural Outpatient Population, *Amer J Dis Child* 113:664–669 (June) 1967.

e. Salmonella-Shigella

780. Alley, R.D., and Pijoan, M.: *Salmonella javiana* Food Infection, *Yale J Biol Med* 15:229–239, 1942.

781. Williams, R.B.: Summary of Salmonella and Shigella of Alaska, *Northwest Med* 49:340–341 (May) 1950.

782. Williams, R.B., and Dodson, M.W.: Salmonella in Alaska, *Public Health Rep* 75:913–916 (Oct) 1960.

783. Elsea, W.R.; Partridge, R.A.; and Neter, E.: Epidemiologic and Microbiological Study of a *Shigella flexneri* Outbreak, *Public Health Rep* 82:347–352 (April) 1967.

784. Wheatley, W., and Van der Veer, J.B., Jr.: A Food-Borne Out-

break of Shigellosis on an Indian Reservation, *Public Health Rep* 84:563–567 (June) 1969.

f. Escherichia coli

785. McAlister, R.; Brody, J.A.; and Overfield, M.: Enteric Disease Due to Enteropathogenic *Escherichia coli* in Hospitalized Infants in Kotzebue, Alaska, *J Pediat* 66:343–348 (Feb) 1965.

786. Brenneman, G., and Fortuine, R.: A Clinical Study of 62 Cases of Diarrhea Associated with Pathogenic *Escherichia coli*, abstracted, *Proc 1st Joint Meet of the Clin Soc and Commissioned Officers Ass USPHS*, Baltimore, Md (May) 1966, p 1.

787. Brenneman, G., and Fortuine, R.: Enteropathogenic *Escherichia coli* Diarrhea in Western Alaska, *Alaska Med* 8:56–63, 1966.

g. Bacterial Meningitis

788. Fortuine, R.: Acute Purulent Meningitis in Alaska Natives: Epidemiology, Diagnosis, and Prognosis, *Canad Med Ass J* 94:19–22 (Jan) 1966.

iv. Tuberculosis

789. Bushnell, G.E.: Study of the Epidemiology of Tuberculosis, New York: Wm. Wood, 1881, p 159.

790. Matthews, W.: Consumption Among the Indians, *Trans Amer Climat Ass*, 1886, pp 234–241.

791. Matthews, W.: Consumption Among the Indians, *NY Med J* 45:1–3, 1887.

792. Mays, T.J.: Does Pulmonary Consumption Tend to Exterminate the American Indian? A Reply to Dr. Washington Matthews, *NY Med J* 46:259, 1887.

793. Matthews, W.: Further Contribution to the Study of Consumption Among the Indians, *Trans Amer Climat Ass*, 1888, pp 136–155.

794. Graham, J.B.: Scrofula Among the Sioux Indians; Its Origin and Nature, *Amer Practitioner News* 9:1–5 (Jan 4) 1890.

795. Bull, H.R.: Tuberculosis Among the Indians, *Colorado State Med Soc Trans*, 1894, pp 314–321.

796. Orton, G.T.: Scrofula Amongst the Indians, *Manitoba and W Canada Lancet* 5:214–215, 1898.

797. Addison, P.: Tuberculosis in Indians, *Canad J Med Surg* (May) 1902.

798. Fox, C.: Tuberculosis Among the Indians of Southeastern Alaska, *Public Health Rep* 16 (pt 2):1615–1616, 1902.

799. Brewer, I.W.: Tuberculosis Among the Indians of Arizona and New Mexico, *NY Med J* 84:981–983, 1906.

800. Walker, J.R.: Tuberculosis Among the Oglala Sioux Indians, *Amer J Med Sci* 122:600–605 (Oct) 1906.

801. Hutchinson, W.: Varieties of Tuberculosis According to Race and Social Condition, *NY Med J* 86:624, 1907.

802. Hrdlička, A.: *Tuberculosis Among Certain Indian Tribes of the United States*, Smithsonian Inst, Bur of Amer Ethnology, Bull 42, 1909, pp 1–48.

803. Klebs, A.C.: *Tuberculosis*, New York: Appleton, 1909, p 127.

804. Murphy, J.A.: *The Prevention of Tuberculosis in Indian Schools*, Natl Ed of US Journal of Proceedings and Addresses, 1909.

805. *Tuberculosis Among Boarding School Pupils*, Dept of Indian Affairs, Canada, Dept Files 140–754, 1909.

806. Brown, W.C.: Disease Among the Aborigines of America and Their Knowledge of Treatment, *Canad J Med Surg* 51:155–158, 1922.

807. *Report of a Committee of the National Tuberculosis Association Appointed on October 28, 1921, on Tuberculosis Among the North American Indians: Tuberculosis Among the North American Indians*, Senate Committee Print, 67th Congress, 4th Session, 1923, p 101.

808. Stone, E.L.: Tuberculosis Among Indians of the Norway House Agency, *Public Health J* 16:76–81, 1925.

809. Collins, R.J., and Leslie, G.L.: Treatment of Tuberculosis Lymphadenitis Among American Indians; Preliminary Report, *Amer Rev Tuberc* 14:646–652, 1926.

810. Cummins, S.L.: Tuberculosis Among Indians of Great Canadian Plains, *Trans Natl Ass Prev Tuberc* 14:85–94, 1928.

811. Ferguson, R.G.: "Tuberculosis Among the Indians of the Great Canadian Plains," in *Transactions of the Fourteenth Annual Conference of the National Association for the Prevention of Tuberculosis*, London: Adlard & Son, 1928, pp 5–56.

812. Ferguson, R.G.: Epidemiology of Tuberculosis in Primitive People, *Edinburgh Med J* 36:199–206, 1929.

813. Maher, S.J.: "Tuberculosis Among the Indians," in *Transactions of the Fifteenth Annual Conference of the National Association for the Prevention of Tuberculosis*, London: Adlard & Son, 1929, pp 95–107; and *Amer Rev Tuberc* 19:407–411, 1929.

814. Abbott, W.A., and Burns, H.A.: Result of Collapse Therapy in an Indian Sanitorium, *Lancet* 52:611–613, 1932.

815. Burns, H.A.: Tuberculosis in the Indian, *Amer Rev Tuberc* 26:498, 506, 1932; and *Amer J Phys Anthrop* 17:442, 1932.

816. Crouch, J.H.: A Study of Tuberculosis Among the Indians in Montana: A Preliminary Report, *Public Health Rep* 47:1907–1914, 1932.

817. Davis, H.: Mantoux Observations in 520 Indian Children, *Nebraska Med J* 17:98–101, 1932.

818. Gillick, D.W.: Social and Community Aspects of the Tuberculosis Problem, *Trans Natl Tuberc Ass* 28:208–212, 1932.

819. Montgomery, L.G.: Tuberculosis Among Indian Children, *Mayo Clin Proc* 7:262–264, 1932.

820. Richards, W.G.: Tuberculosis Among the Indians in Montana, *Amer Rev Tuberc* 26:492–515, 1932.

821. Ringle, O.F.; Feldman, F.F.; and Burns, H.A.: Tuberculosis Survey in an Indian County in Minnesota, 1931–32, *Lancet* 52:538–539, 1932.

822. Warner, H.J.: Incidence of Tuberculosis Infection Among School Children on Five Montana Reservations, *Amer Rev Tuberc* 26:507–515, 1932.

823. Ferguson, R.G.: The Indian Tuberculosis Problem and Some Preventive Measures, *Trans Natl Tuberc Ass* 29:93–106, 1933.

824. Montgomery, L.G.: Tuberculosis Among Pupils of a Canadian School for Indians, *Amer Rev Tuberc* 28:502–515, 1933.

825. Fellows, F.S.: Mortality in the Native Races of the Territory

of Alaska, with Special Reference to Tuberculosis, *Public Health Rep* 49:289–298, 1934.

826. Ferguson, R.G.: Tuberculosis Problems and Some Preventive Measures, *Canad Med Ass J* 30:544–547, 1934.

827. Simes, A.B., and Paynter, L.E.: Occurrence of Virulent Tubercle Bacilli in Excreta of Tuberculous Children, *Tubercle* 15:498–503, 1934.

828. Stewart, D.A.: Indians and Tuberculosis, *Ninette*, Manitoba, 1934.

829. Aronson, J.D.: Incidence of Tuberculous Infection in Some Rural Communities in Michigan, *Amer J Hyg* 21:543–561, 1935.

830. Long, E.R.: Rise and Fall of Tuberculosis in Certain American Peoples, *Puerto Rico J Public Health Trop Med* 10:270–287, 1935.

831. Walton, C.H.A.: A Study of the Racial Incidence of Tuberculosis in the Province of Manitoba, *Amer Rev Tuberc* 32:183–195, 1935.

832. Gilbert, M.E.: Occupational Therapy Program at Choctaw-Chickasaw Sanitorium, *Occup Therapy* 15:109–116, 1936.

833. Korns, J.H.: Comparative Tuberculosis Findings Among Indians and White Persons in Cattaraugus County, New York, *Amer Rev Tuberc* 34:550–560, 1936.

834. Long, E.R., and Hetherington, H.W.: A Tuberculosis Survey in the Papago Indian Area of Southern Arizona, *Amer Rev Tuberc* 33 (suppl):407–433 (March) 1936.

835. Stewart, D.A.: Red Man and White Plague, *Canad Med Ass J* 35:674–676, 1936.

836. Toone, W.M.: Seeking Tuberculosis with Aid of a Microscope, *Canad Med Ass J* 35:191, 1936.

837. Long, E.R.: Brief Comparison of Tuberculosis in White, Indian, and Negro Races, *Amer Rev Tuberc* 35:1–5, 1937.

838. Carswell, J.A.: Poverty and Tuberculosis, with Particular Reference to Economic and Social Significance of High Death Rates Among Alaskans, *Trans Natl Tuberc Ass* 34:233–246, 1938.

839. Rider, A.S.: Anti-Tuberculosis Work at Flandreau Indian School, *J Lancet* 58:175–177, 1938.

840. Ross, E.L., and Paine, A.L.: Tuberculosis Survey of Manitoba Indians, *Canad Med Ass J* 41:180–184, 1939.

841. Alley, R.: Tuberculosis Among Indians, *Dis Chest* 6:44–50, 1940.

842. Aronson, J.D.; Parr, E.I.; and Saylor, R.M.: BCG (Calmette-Guérin) Vaccine; Local Reaction to Injection, *Amer Rev Tuberc* 42:651–666, 1940.

843. Jones, L.R.: Tuberculosis on a Small Thickly Populated Indian Reservation, *Amer Rev Tuberc* 42:197–202, 1940.

844. Moore, P.E.: Tuberculosis Control in the Indian Population of Canada, *Canad J Public Health* 32:13–17, 1941.

845. Townsend, J.G., et al: Tuberculosis Control Among the North American Indians, *Trans 37th Ann Meet of the Natl Tuberc Ass*, 1941, pp 41–52.

846. Townsend, J.G., et al: Tuberculosis Control Among the North American Indians, *Amer Rev Tuberc* 45:41–52, 1942.

847. Townsend, J.G., et al: Tuberculosis in the North American Indian, *Proc Amer Scientific Congress, 1940,* 6:261–267, 1942.

848. Pijoan, M., and Sedlacek, B.: Ascorbic Acid in Tuberculous Navajo Indians, *Amer Rev Tuberc* 48:342–346, 1943.

849. McGibony, J.R., and Dahlstrom, A.W.: Tuberculosis Among Montana Indians, *Amer Rev Tuberc* 52:104–121, 1945.

850. Aronson, J.D., and Palmer, C.E.: Experience with BCG Vaccine in the Control of Tuberculosis Among North American Indians, *Public Health Rep* 61:802–820 (June) 1946.

851. BCG Vaccination Against Tuberculosis, *Public Health Rep* 61:801 (June) 1946.

852. Aronson, J.D., and Palmer, C.E.: Calmette-Guérin Immunization in the Control of Tuberculosis Among North American Indians, *Bol Med Social (Sanitago)* 14:226–237, 1947.

853. McMinimy, D.J.: Preliminary Report on Tuberculosis Incidence in Alaska, *Alaska's Health* 5:4–5 (Oct) 1947.

854. Myers, J.A., and Dustin, U.L.: Albert Reifel and Tuberculosis Among the Indians, *Hygeia* 25:272, 1947.

855. Aronson, J.D.: BCG Vaccination Among American Indians, *Amer Rev Tuberc* 57:96–99 (Jan) 1948.

856. Aronson, J.D.: Protective Vaccination Against Tuberculosis

with Special Reference to BCG Vaccination, *Amer Rev Tuberc* 58:255–281 (Sept) 1948.

857. Van Hagen, G.E.: Alaska's Time Bomb—TB, *Alaska Life* 11:12–13, 22, 1948.

858. Ferguson, R.G., and Simes, A.B.: BCG (Calmette-Guérin) Vaccination of Indian Infants in Saskatchewan, *Tubercle* 30:5–11, 1949.

859. McDougall, J.B.: *Tuberculosis: A Global Study in Social Pathology*, Baltimore, Md: Williams and Wilkins, 1949, p 242.

860. Reifel, A.: Tuberculosis Among Indians of the United States, *Dis Chest* 16:234–247 (Aug) 1949.

861. Tuberculosis Among American Indians, editorial, *Dis Chest* 16:248–249 (Aug) 1949.

862. DeLien, H., and Dahlstrom, A.W.: Tuberculosis Control Among American Indians, *J Lancet* 70:131–134 (April) 1950.

863. T.B. Hospital for Alaska Designed for Conversion, *Architectural Rec* 108:160, 162, 1950.

864. DeLien, H.: Continuity in Program—Necessity in Tuberculosis Control Among American Indians, *J Lancet* 71:136–137 (April) 1951.

865. DeLien, H., and Dahlstrom, A.W.: Ethnic Reservoir of Tuberculosis, *Amer J Public Health* 41:528–532 (May) 1951.

866. Gaumand, E., and Therrier, E.: Indians and Tuberculosis of the Skin and Bones, *Canad Med Ass J* 64:122–126 (Feb) 1951.

867. Tuberculosis Survey: James and Hudson Bays, 1950, *Arctic Circle* 4:45–47 (March) 1951.

868. Aronson, J.D., and Aronson, C.F.: Appraisal of Protective Value of BCG Vaccine, *JAMA* 149:334–343 (May) 1952.

869. Dubois, R., and Dubois, J.: *The White Plague*, Boston: Little Brown & Co, 1952.

870. Foard, F.T.: The Tuberculosis Problem Among Indians, *Trans 48th Ann Meet of the Natl Tuberc Ass* 48:787–794, 1952.

871. Aronson, J.D., and Aronson, C.F.: The Correlation of the Tuberculin Reaction with Roentgenographically Demonstrable Pulmonary Lesions in BCG-Vaccinated and Control Persons, *Amer Rev Tuberc* 68:713–726 (Nov) 1953.

872. Blomquist, E.T., and Weiss, E.S.: The Tuberculosis Problem in the Pacific Territories: Alaska, *Trans Natl Ass Stud Tuberc* 49:46–49, 1953.

873. Davis, R., and Salsbury, C.G.: Health and Tuberculosis Problems Among Indians, *Trans Natl Ass Stud Tuberc* 49:479–487, 1953.

874. Leggett, E.A.: Outpatient Services for Tuberculous Indians in Minnesota, *J Lancet* 73:127–129, 154 (April) 1953.

875. Paul, F.L.: *Home Care of the Tuberculous in Alaska,* US Dept of Interior, Indian Serv, Alaska Native Serv, 1953, p 115.

876. Stein, S.C., and Aronson, J.D.: The Occurrence of Pulmonary Lesions in BCG-Vaccinated and Unvaccinated Persons, *Amer Rev Tuberc* 68:695–712 (Nov) 1953.

877. Vaccinations Against TB given to 2,486 Alaskans in Past Year; Vaccine Given in 41 Kenai-to-Barrow Villages, *Alaska's Health* 10:1–2 (June) 1953.

878. Weiss, E.S.: Tuberculin Sensitivity in Alaska, *Public Health Rep* 68:23–27 (Jan) 1953.

879. Anchorage Medical Center Admits First TB Patients Immediately After Opening; Alaska Native Service Hospital Has 300 TB and 100 General Beds, *Alaska's Health* 11:1, 4 (Feb) 1954.

880. Caron, M.: First Results of Use of Isoniazid, Streptomycin & PAS With or Without Collapse Therapy in a Group of Adult Indians and Eskimos and Boys with Pulmonary Tuberculosis, *Union Med Canada* 83:883–893, 1954.

881. New ANS Anchorage Medical Center Brings Tuberculosis Beds in Territory to 820; History Shows that TB Hospitals Developed Very Slowly in Alaska, *Alaska's Health* 11:2 (Feb) 1954.

882. Thomas, G.W.: Pulmonary Tuberculosis in Northern Newfoundland and Labrador, *N Eng J Med* 251:374–377 (Sept) 1954.

883. Aronson, J.D., and Taylor, H.C.: The Trend of Tuberculous Infection Among Some Indian Tribes and the Influence of BCG Vaccination on the Tuberculin Test, *Amer Rev Tuberc* 72:35–52 (July) 1955.

884. Hayman, C.R.: The Problem of Tuberculosis from a Terri-

torial Health Standpoint, abstracted, *Sci in Alaska,* Proc 6th
Alaskan Sci Conf (1955), AAAS, Alaska Div, pp 134–135.

885. *Tuberculosis Services in Canada,* Canad Dept of Natl Health
and Welfare, Res Div, Memo 11, 1955, p 65.

886. Williams, R.B.: A Study of the Types of Tuberculosis in
Alaska, *Arctic* 8:215–233, 1955.

887. Project to Combat Tuberculosis in Indians, editorial, *Public
Health Rep* 71:394 (April) 1956.

888. *Tuberculosis Among Indians and Eskimos, 1950–52,* Canad
Bur of Statis, Ottawa: Queens Printer, 1956.

889. Lear, L.: Chemotherapy in Alaska, *Amer J Nurs* 57:320–322
(March) 1957.

890. Aronson, J.D.; Aronson, C.F.; and Taylor, H.C.: A Twenty-
Year Appraisal of BCG Vaccination in the Control of Tuberculosis, *Arch Intern Med* 101:881–893 (May) 1958.

891. Beamish, W.E.: Renal Tuberculosis in a Native Population,
Canad Med Ass J 81:238–241 (Aug 15) 1959.

892. Deuschle, K.W.: Tuberculosis Among the Navajo, *Amer Rev
Resp Dis* 80:200–206 (Aug) 1959.

893. Gentles, E.W.: Tuberculosis in Alaska, *Alaska Med* 1:53–54,
1959.

894. Lane, R.F.: A Two- to Nine-Year Survey of Chest Surgery for
Pulmonary Tuberculosis in British Columbia Indians, *Dis
Chest* 35:629–633 (June) 1959.

895. Comstock, G.W., and Porter, M.E.: "Tuberculin Sensitivity
in Natives of the Lower Yukon and Its Relation to Tuberculosis," in *Sci in Alaska,* Proc 9th Alaskan Sci Conf (1958),
AAAS, Alaska Div, 1960, pp 116–119.

896. Deuschle, K.W.: Tuberculosis Among the Navajo Indians,
Penn Med J 63:304–305, 1960.

897. Levinson, R.A., and Cummings, M.M.: A Study of Tuberculin
Reactions in an Indian Hospital Population, abstracted, *J Clin
Invest* 39:1005–1006 (June) 1960.

898. Mead, P.A.: Intracranial Tuberculomas—Experience with the
Alaska Native Health Service, Anchorage: 1954–59, *Alaska
Med* 2:69–75, 1960.

899. Comstock, G.W., and Philip, R.N.: Decline of the Tubercu-

losis Epidemic in Alaska, *Public Health Rep* 76:19–24 (Jan) 1961.

900. Moore, P.E.: No Longer Captain: A History of Tuberculosis and Its Control Amongst Canadian Indians, *Canad Med J* 84:1012–1016 (May 5) 1961.

901. Phillips, F.J.: A Preliminary Report of Out-Patient Treatment of Pulmonary Tuberculosis, *Alaska Med* 3:1–4, 1961.

902. Sievers, M.L.: The Second Great Imitator—Tuberculosis, *JAMA* 176:809–810 (June) 1961.

903. Silva, J.A.: Can Tuberculosis Among Indians Be Eradicated? *Oklahoma J Public Health* 4:15–16, 1961.

904. Winter, L.H.: Increase in Tuberculosis Is Noted, *Alaska Health Welfare* 18:1–2 (Oct) 1961.

905. Comstock, G.W.: Isoniazid Prophylaxis in an Undeveloped Area, *Amer Rev Resp Dis* 86:810–823 (Dec) 1962.

906. Phillips, F.J.: The Tuberculosis Problem in Alaska, *Alaska Med* 4:101–102, 1962.

907. Porter, M.E., and Comstock, G.W.: Ambulatory Chemotherapy in Alaska, *Public Health Rep* 77:1021–1032 (Dec) 1962.

908. Ross, C.A.; Dafoe, C.S.; and Nicholson, M.W.: Pulmonary Resection for Tuberculosis, *Canad J Surg* 5:259–264 (July) 1962.

909. Thomas, G.W.: The Decline and Fall of Pulmonary Tuberculosis in Northern Newfoundland and Labrador, *Among the Deep Sea Fishers* 60:3–4 (April) 1962.

910. Whaley, H.S.: Status of Childhood Tuberculosis in Alaska, *Alaska Med* 4:46–48, 1962.

911. Armstrong, F.B., and Edwards, A.M.: Intracranial Tuberculoma in Native Races of Canada: With Special Reference to Symptomatic Epilepsy and Neurologic Features, *Canad Med Ass J* 89:56–65 (July) 1963.

912. Paine, A.L., and Matwichuk, Z.: Five to Seventeen Year-End Results in 402 Patients with Pulmonary Resection for Tuberculosis, *Amer Rev Resp Dis* 90:760–770 (Nov) 1964.

913. Fraser, R.I.: Alaska Tuberculosis Rate Shows Decline But Is Rising Again, *Alaska Health Welfare* 22:4–5 (April) 1965.

914. Fraser, R.I.: "Tuberculosis Control in Alaska," in *Sci in Alaska,*

Proc 16th Alaskan Sci Conf (1965), AAAS, Alaska Div, 1965, pp 48–54.

915. Fraser, R.I.: Tuberculosis in Alaska in 1965, *Alaska Med* 7:12–15, 1965.

916. Gaenslen, E.C.: Tuberculous Meningitis Among Alaskan Natives, *Alaska Med* 7:16–18, 1965.

917. Lifschitz, M.: The Value of the Tuberculin Skin Test as a Screening Test for Tuberculosis Among BCG-Vaccinated Children, *Pediatrics* 36:624–627 (Oct) 1965.

918. Omran, R., and Deuschle, K.W.: A Controlled Evaluation of a Selective Method of Tuberculosis-Case Finding, *Amer Rev Resp Dis* 91:215–224 (Feb) 1965.

919. Matas, M.: Tuberculosis Programs of the Medical Services, Dept. of National Health and Welfare, *Med Serv J Canad* 22:878–883, 1966.

920. Wrigley, J., and Diddams, A.: The Status of Urinary Tuberculosis Among the Alaska Native Population Since 1953, abstracted, *Proc 1st Joint Meet of the Clin Soc and Commissioned Officers Ass USPHS*, Baltimore, Md (May) 1966, p 25.

921. Wallace, H.M.: Childhood Tuberculosis with Reference to the American Indian, *Public Health Rep* 82:3–34 (Jan) 1967.

922. Edwards, L.B.; Comstock, G.W.; and Palmer, C.E.: Contributions of Northern Populations to the Understanding of Tuberculin Sensitivity, *Arch Environ Health* 17:507–516 (Oct) 1968.

923. Flood, F., and Templin, D.: Control of an Epidemic of Tuberculosis in an Indian Boarding School, abstracted, *Proc 3rd Joint Meet of the Clin Soc and Commissioned Officers Ass USPHS*, San Francisco, Calif (March) 1968, p 7.

924. Hanson, M.L., and Comstock, G.W.: Efficacy of Hydrocortisone Ointment in the Treatment of Local Reactions to Tuberculin Skin Tests, *Amer Rev Resp Dis* 97:472–473 (March) 1968.

925. Robinson, C.L.N.: Pulmonary Resection for Tuberculosis in Saskatchewan, 1959–1966, *Dis Chest* 53:288–293 (March) 1968.

926. Shoop, J.D.: The Use of the Routine Apical Lordotic Chest Film in the Investigation of Populations with High Risk of

Pulmonary Tuberculosis, abstracted, *Proc 3rd Joint Meet of the Clin Soc and Commissioned Officers Ass USPHS*, San Francisco, Calif (March) 1968, p 7.

v. Syphilis

927. Pousma, R.H.: Venereal Diseases Among Navajos, *Southwest Med* 13:503–505, 1929.
928. Cark, W.: *Syphilis in New Mexico*, N Mexico Tuberc Ass, Santa Fe, NM, 1934.
929. Shattuck, G.C.: Lesions of Syphilis in American Indians, *Amer J Trop Med* 18:577–586, 1938.
930. McCammon, C.S.; Dufner, F.J.; and Felsman, F.W.: Syphilis Among the Navajo Indians, *J Vener Dis Inform* 32:28–33, 1951.
931. Orr, H., and Rentiers, R.L.: Study of Syphilis in Northern Alberta, *Arch Derm* 63:85–90 (Jan) 1951.
932. DeLien, H., and Hadley, J.N.: Venereal Disease Problem Among North American Indians, *J Lancet* 72:513–515 (Nov) 1952.
933. Outbreak of Early Infectious Syphilis in the Black Hills and Pine Ridge Indian Reservation of South Dakota, January–April, 1962, *S Dakota J Med Pharm* 15:390–391 (Oct) 1962.

vi. Amebiasis

934. Eaton, R.D.P.: Amebiasis in Saskatchewan, *Canad J Public Health* 56:483–486 (Nov) 1965.
935. Meerovitch, E., and Eaton, R.D.P.: Outbreak of Amebiasis Among Indians in Northwestern Saskatchewan, Canada, *Amer J Trop Med* 14:719–723 (Sept) 1965.
936. Buchan, D.J.: Amebiasis in Northern Saskatchewan: Clinical Aspects, *Canad Med Ass J* 99:683–687 (Oct) 1968.
937. Eaton, R.D.P.: Amebiasis in Northern Saskatchewan: Epidemiological Considerations, *Canad Med Ass J* 99:709–711 (Oct) 1968.
938. Miller, M.J.; Mathews, W.H.; and Moore, D.F.: Amebiasis in Northern Saskatchewan: Pathological Aspects, *Canad Med Ass J* 99:969–705 (Oct) 1968.

939. Tchang, S.: Amebiasis in Northern Saskatchewan: Radiological Aspects, *Canad Med Ass J* 99:688–695 (Oct) 1968.

vii. Helminth Infestations

940. Healy, G.R., et al: Intestinal Parasites of Cherokee Indian School Children with Special Reference to Ascariasis and Amebiasis, abstracted, *Proc 1st Joint Meet of the Clin Soc and Commissioned Officers Ass USPHS*, Baltimore, Md (May) 1966, p 4.
941. Becker, D.A.: Enteric Parasites of Indians and Anglo-Americans, Chiefly on the Winnebago and Omaha Reservations in Nebraska, II: Pinworms in Indians on the Winnebago and Omaha Reservations, *Nebraska Med J* 53:347–349 (July) 1968.
942. Healy, G.R., et al: Prevalence of Ascariasis and Amebiasis in Cherokee Indian School Children, *Public Health Rep* 84:907–914 (Oct) 1969.

D. DISEASES TRANSMITTED FROM ANIMALS, ANIMAL PRODUCTS, OR SOIL TO MAN

i. Zoonoses in General

943. Rausch, R.L.: Animal-Borne Diseases, *Public Health Rep* 68: 533–534 (May) 1953.
944. Rausch, R.L.: Animal-Borne Diseases in Alaska and Their Public Health Significance, *Proc Intl Veterinary Congress* (*Stockholm*) 8:254–259, 1953.
945. Rausch, R.L.: "A Summary of Current Information on Some Animal-Borne Diseases in Alaska," in *Sci in Alaska*, Proc 3rd Alaskan Sci Conf (1952), AAAS, Alaska Div, 1954, pp 144–147.
946. Rausch, R.L.: "A Review of Zoonotic Diseases of Special Importance in Subarctic and Arctic Regions," Doc 9 in *Conf on Med and Public Health in the Arctic and Antarctic*, WHO, Geneva, 1962, p 10.
947. Rausch, R.L.: Zoonotic Diseases in the Changing Arctic, *Arch Environ Health* 17:627–630 (Oct) 1968.

948. Hildes, J.A.: Some Zoonotic Problems in the Canadian Arctic, *Arch Environ Health* 18:133–137 (Jan) 1969.

ii. Viral

949. Solman, V.E.F.: An Outbreak of Rabies in Northwest Canada, 1951–1952, *Arctic Circle* 5:57, 1952.
950. Wilt, J.C.; Hildes, J.A.; and Stanfield, F.S.: The Prevalence of Complement-Fixing Antibodies Against Psittacosis in the Canadian Arctic, *Canad Med Ass J* 81:731–733 (Nov) 1959.
951. Work, T.H.: Serological Evidence of Arbovirus Infection in the Seminole Indians of Southern Florida, *Science* 2:270–272 (July) 1964.

iii. Rickettsial

952. Herbert, F.A., et al: Q Fever in Alberta—Infection in Humans and Animals, *Canad Med Ass J* 93:1207–1210, 1965.

iv. Bacterial

a. Plague

953. Allen, G.: Recent Human Plague in the U.S., abstracted, *Proc 1st Joint Meet of the Clin Soc and Commissioned Officers Ass USPHS*, Baltimore, Md (May) 1966, p 28.
954. Kartman, L.; Goldenberg, M.I.; and Hubbert, W.T.: Recent Observations on the Epidemiology of Plague in the United States, *Amer J Public Health* 56:1554 (Sept) 1966.
955. Collins, R.N., et al: Plague Epidemic in New Mexico, 1965, *Public Health Rep* 82:1077–1099 (Dec) 1967.
956. Kartman, L., et al: Plague Epidemic in New Mexico, 1965: Epidemiologic Features and Results of Field Studies, *Public Health Rep* 82:1084–1094 (Dec) 1967.
957. Martin, A.R., et al: Plague Meningitis: A Report of 3 Cases in Children and Review of the Problem, *Pediatrics* 40:610–615 (Oct) 1967.
958. The Navajos' Way of Life Exposes Them to Plague, *Public Health Rep* 82:219 (March) 1967.

959. Tirador, D.F., et al: An Emergency Program to Control Plague, *Public Health Rep* 82:1094–1099 (March) 1967.

b. Tularemia

960. Philip, C.B.: Tularaemia in Alaska, *Proc Pacif Sci Conf* (*6th*), 5:71–73, 1942.

961. Williams, R.B.: Tularaemia in Alaska, *Alaska's Health* 3:2–3, 1943.

962. Williams, R.B.: Tularemia: First Case To Be Reported in Alaska, *Public Health Rep* 61:875–876 (June) 1946.

963. MacKinnon, A.G.: Pulmonary Type of Tularaemia (Two Cases), *Canad Med Ass J* 56:541–542 (May) 1947.

964. Philip, C.B.; Gill, G.D.; and Geary, J.M.: Notes on the Rabbit Tick *Haemaphysalis leporis-palustris* (Packard), and Tularaemia in Central Alaska, *J Parasit* 40:484–485 (Aug) 1954.

965. Grumbles, L.C.: "Serological Evidence of Tularemia in Man in Alaska," in *Sci in Alaska*, Proc 6th Alaskan Sci Conf (1955), AAAS, Alaska Div, pp 133–134.

966. Hopla, C.E.: *Epidemiology of Tularemia*, US Arctic Aeromedical Lab, Ladd Air Force Base, Techn Rep 59–1, 1960, p 42.

967. Hopla, C.E.: Observations on the Natural History of Tularemia in Central Alaska, abstracted, *Sci in Alaska*, Proc 12th Alaskan Sci Conf (1961), AAAS, Alaska Div, 1962, pp 185–186.

968. Philip, R.N., et al: Serologic and Skin Test Evidence of Tularemia Infection Among Alaskan Eskimos, Indians, and Aleuts, *J Infect Dis* 110:220–230 (May–June) 1962.

969. Saliba, G., et al: An Outbreak of Human Tularemia Associated with the American Dog Tick, *Dermacentor variabilis*, *Amer J Trop Med* 15:531 (July) 1966.

c. Brucellosis

970. Huntley, B.E.; Philip, R.N.; and Maynard, J.E.: Survey of Brucellosis in Alaska, *J Infect Dis* 112:100–106 (Jan–Feb) 1963.

v. Fungal

971. Aronson, J.D.; Saylor, R.M.; and Parr, E.I.: Relationship of Coccidioidomycosis to Calcified Pulmonary Nodules, *Arch Path* 34:31–48, 1942.

972. Moore, M., and Mantling, G.: Sporotrichosis Following Mosquito Bite; Description of Lesions in Girl of Indian and French Descent, *Arch Derm Syph* 48:525–526, 1943.

973. Comstock, G.W.: Histoplasmin Sensitivity in Alaskan Natives, *Amer Rev Tuberc* 79:542 (April) 1959.

974. Sievers, M.L.: Coccidioidomycosis Among Southwestern American Indians, *Amer Rev Resp Dis* 90:920–926 (Dec) 1964.

975. Carlile, W.K.: Disseminated Coccidioidomycosis in the American Indians, abstracted, *Proc 1st Joint Meet of the Clin Soc and Commissioned Officers Ass USPHS*, Baltimore, Md (May) 1966, p 29.

vi. Malarial

976. Woodward: The Nez-Perce on the Indian Reservation Being Destroyed by Malaria, *Gaillards' Med J* 37:225, 1884.

977. St. Childs, J.R.: *Malaria—Colonization in the Carolina Low Country, 1526–1696,* Johns Hopkins U Studies in History and Political Sci, Ser 58, Baltimore, Md: Johns Hopkins Press, 1940.

978. Levine, N.D.: *Malaria in the Interior Valley of North America* (abridgement of book by Daniel Drake, 1850), Urbana: U of Ill Press, 1964.

979. Giglioli, G.: "Malaria in the American Indian," in *Biomedical Challenges Presented by the American Indian,* WHO, Pan American Health Org, Publ 165, 1968, pp 104–113.

vii. Helminth Infestations

a. Echinococcosis (Hydatid Disease)

980. Rausch, R.L.: Hydatid Disease in Boreal Regions, *Arctic* 5: 157–174, 1952.

981. Sweatman, G.K.: Distribution and Incidence of *Echinococcus granulosa* in Man and Other Animals with Special Reference to Canada, *Canad J Public Health* 43:480–486, 1952.

982. Miller, M.J.: Hydatid Infection in Canada, *Canad Med Ass J* 68:423 (May) 1953.

983. Coddington, F.L., and Moore, P.H.: "Echinococcus Cysts in Human Beings," in *Sci in Alaska,* Proc 3rd Alaskan Sci Conf (1952), AAAS, Alaska Div, 1954, pp 147–149.

984. Meltzer, H.L., et al: Echinococcosis in North American Indians and Eskimos, *Canad Med Ass J* 75:121–128 (July) 1956.

985. Poole, J.B., and Wolfgang, R.W.: Hydatid Disease in the Yukon and Northwest Territories, abstracted, *Canad J Public Health* 47:44 (Jan) 1956.

986. Wolfgang, R.W., and Poole, J.B.: Distribution of *Echinococcus* Disease in Northwestern Canada, *Amer J Trop Med* 5:869–871 (Sept) 1956.

987. Davis, T.R.A.: Hydatid Disease in Alaska, *Amer J Med* 23:99 (July) 1957.

988. Poole, J.B.: Echinococcus Disease in Northern North America, *Amer J Trop Med* 6:424 (May) 1957.

989. West, J.T.: Malignant Echinococcus Disease of the Liver, *Alaska Med* 1:107–114, 1959.

990. Cameron, T.W.M.: The Incidence and Diagnosis of Hydatid Cyst in Canada: *Echinococcus granulosus* Var. *Canadensis, Parasitologia* 2:381–390, 1960.

991. Rausch, R.L.: Recent Studies on Hydatid Disease in Alaska, *Parasitologia* 2:391–398, 1960.

b. Trichinosis

992. Brown, M., et al: A Note on Trichinosis in Animals of the Canadian Northwest Territories, *Canad J Public Health* 40:20–21 (Dec) 1949.

c. Diphyllobothriasis

993. Babero, B.B.: "Diphyllobothriasis in Alaska," in *Sci in Alaska,*

Proc 2nd Alaskan Sci Conf (1951), AAAS, Alaska Div, pp 312–314.

994. Wolfgang, R.W.: Indian and Eskimo Diphyllobothriasis, *Canad Med Ass J* 70:536–539 (May) 1954.

VI. NEOPLASMS

995. Levin, I.: Cancer Among the American Indians and Its Bearing upon the Ethnological Distribution of the Disease, *Z Krebsforsch* 9:422–435, 1910.

996. Hoffman, F.L.: *Cancer Among North American Indians, the Health Progress of the North American Indian, the Indian as a Life Insurance Risk*, Newark, NJ: Prudential Press, 1928, p 85.

997. Lee, B.J.: El Cancer Entre los Indios del Suroeste, *Bol Liga Contra Cancer* 1:234–241, 1930.

998. Lee, B.J.: The Incidence of Cancer Among the Indians in the Southwest, *Surg Gynec Obstet* 50:196–199, 1930.

999. Palmer, E.P.: Cancer Among the Indians of the United States, with an Analysis of Cancer in Arizona, *Southwest Med* 22:483–487 (Dec) 1938.

1000. Courville, C.B., and Abbott, K.H.: Pathology of Cranial Tumors; Metastatic Tumors of the Calvarium, with Incidental Reference to Their Occurrence in American Aborigines, *Bull Los Angeles Neurol Soc* 10:129–154, 1945.

1001. Palmer, E.P.: Incidence of Cancer Among Indians of the United States and Canada, with Specific Reference to Arizona, *Acta Un Int Cancr* 9:373–391, 1953.

1002. Warwick, O.H., and Phillips, A.J.: Cancer Among Canadian Indians, *Brit J Cancer* 8:223–230, 1954.

1003. Phillips, A.J.: Cancer Among Canadian Indians, *Schweiz Z Allg Path* 18:500–506, 1955.

1004. Lawson, R.N.; Saunders, A.L.; and Cowen, R.D.: Breast Cancer and Heptaldehyde (Preliminary Report), *Canad Med Ass J* 75:486–488 (Sept) 1956.

1005. Salsbury, C.G.: Cancer Immunity in the Navajo, *Arizona Med* 13:309–310 (Aug) 1956.

1006. Smith, R.L.; Salsbury, C.G.; and Gilliam, A.G.: Recorded and Expected Mortality Among the Navajo, with Special Reference to Cancer, *J Natl Cancer Inst* 17:77–89 (July) 1956.

1007. Smith, R.L.: Recorded and Expected Mortality Among the Indians of the United States, with Special Reference to Cancer, *J Natl Cancer Inst* 18:385–396 (March) 1957.

1008. Salsbury, C.G., et al: A Cancer Detection Survey of Carcinoma of the Lung and Female Pelvis Among Navajos of the Navajo Indian Reservation, *Surg Gynec Obstet* 108:257–266 (March) 1959.

1009. Carcinoma in Blackfoot Indians, *Public Health Rep* 75:651 (July) 1960.

1010. Stefansson, V.: *Cancer: Disease of Civilization? An Anthropological and Historical Study,* New York: Hill and Wang, 1960, p 180.

1011. Sievers, M.L., and Cohen, S.L.: Lung Cancer Among Indians of the Southwestern United States, *Ann Intern Med* 54:912–915 (May) 1961.

1012. Thomas, G.W.: Carcinoma Among Labrador Eskimos and Indians, *Canad J Surg* 4:465–468 (July) 1961.

1013. Bivens, M.D., et al: Carcinoma of the Cervix in the Indians of the Southwest, *Amer J Obstet Gynec* 83:1203–1207 (May) 1962.

1014. Torrey, E.F.: Malignant Neoplasm Among Alaskan Natives: An Epidemiological Approach to Cancer, *McGill Med J* 31:107–115 (Oct) 1962.

1015. Justice, J.W.: Cancer Screening Program, *Alaska Med* 6:106–110, 1964.

1016. Johnson, M.W.: "Lung Cancer Among the Alaska Natives," in *Sci in Alaska,* Proc 15th Alaskan Sci Conf (1964), AAAS, Alaska Div, 1965, pp 110–114.

1017. Sheehan, J.F.: Carcinoma of the Cervix in Indian Women, *Nebraska Med J* 50:553–558, 1965.

1018. Jaffe, B.: Incidence of Maxillary Cancer in the Navajo Indians, abstracted, *Proc 2nd Joint Meet of the Clin Soc and*

Commissioned Officers Ass USPHS, Atlanta, Ga (May) 1967, p 19.

1019. Boggs, D.C., and McMahon, L.J.: Hand-Schüller-Christian Disease Presenting as Gingivitis, *Oral Surg* 26:261–264 (Aug) 1968.

1020. Barton, S.: Mucocoele of the Frontal Sinus—Report of a Case in a Southwestern Indian, abstracted, *Proc 4th Joint Meet of the Clin Soc and Commissioned Officers Ass USPHS*, Boston (June) 1969.

1021. Jordan, S.W., et al: Carcinoma of the Cervix in American Indian Women, *Cancer* 23:1227–1232 (May) 1969.

VII. MENTAL HEALTH AND PSYCHIATRIC DISORDERS

A. MENTAL HEALTH AND HYGIENE

1022. McKenzie, F.A.: The Assimilation of the American Indian, *Amer J Sociol* 19:761–772, 1914.

1023. Parker, A.C.: The Social Elements of the Indian Problems, *Amer J Sociol* 22:252–267, 1916.

1024. McCaskill, J.C.: Social Hygiene in Racial Problems, *J Soc Hyg* 18:438–446, 1932.

1025. Hallowell, A.I.: Culture and Mental Disorder, *J Abnorm Soc Psychol* 29:1–9, 1934.

1026. Anderson, F.N.: Mental Hygiene Survey of Problem Children in Oklahoma, *Ment Hyg* 20:472–476, 1936.

1027. Devereux, G.: The Mental Hygiene of the American Indian, *Ment Hyg* 26:71–84, 1942.

1028. Spitzer, A.: Social Disorganization Among the Montana Blackfeet, *Amer Cath Soc Rev* 11:218–233, 1950.

1029. Lantis, M.: *Acculturation and Health* (rev Feb 1963), from Pittsburgh U Grad Sch of Public Health: *Alaska's Health, A Survey Report*, Pittsburgh, Pa, 1954, chap 2.

1030. Willis, J.S.: Mental Health in the North, *Med Serv J Canada* 16:689, 1960.

1031. Hoyt, E.E.: Young Indians: Some Problems and Issues of Mental Hygiene, *Ment Hyg* 46:41–47 (Jan) 1962.

1032. Pankow, G.: The Body Image in a Hopi Indian, *J Psychosom Med* 8:223–225 (July–Sept) 1962.

1033. Willis, J.S., and Martin, M.: "Mental Health in Canada's North," Doc 26 in *Conf on Med and Public Health in the Arctic and Antarctic*, WHO, Geneva, 1962, p 25.

1034. Krush, T.P., and Bjork, J.: Mental Health Factors in an Indian Boarding School, *Ment Hyg* 49:94–103 (Jan) 1965.

1035. Henderson, N.E.: Cross Cultural Action Research: Some Limitations, Advantages, and Problems, *J Soc Psychol* 73:61–70 (Oct) 1967.

1036. Gaddes, W.H., et al: Psychomotor Intelligence and Spatial Imagery in Two Northwest Indian and Two White Groups of Children, *J Soc Psychol* 75:35–42 (Jan) 1968.

1037. Leighton, A.H.: The Mental Health of the American Indian, *Amer J Psychiat* 125:217–218 (Aug) 1968.

1038. Leighton, A.H.: The Therapeutic Process in Cross Cultural Perspective—A Symposium: Fragments from a Navajo Ceremonial, *Amer J Psychiat* 124:1176–1178 (March) 1968.

1039. Leon, R.G.: The Mental Health of the American Indian: Some Implications for a Preventive Program for American Indians, *Amer J Psychiat* 125:232–236 (Aug) 1968.

1040. *The Mental Health of the American Indian* (a symposium at the 123rd Ann Meet of the Amer Psychiat Ass, Detroit, May 8–12, 1967), 125:113–132 (July) 1968.

1041. Williamson, R.G.: The Canadian Arctic, Sociocultural Change, *Arch Environ Health* 17:484–491 (Oct) 1968.

1042. Cocking, R.R.: Fantasy Confession Among Arapaho Indian Children, *J Genet Psychol* 114:229–235 (Jan) 1969.

1043. Johnson, D.G.: Conference on Increasing Representation in Medical Schools of Afro-Americans, Mexican-Americans, and American Indians, *J Med Educ* 114:710–711 (Aug) 1969.

1044. Mickelson, N.I., et al: Cumulative Language Deficit Among Indian Children, *Exceptional Child* 36:187–190 (Nov) 1969.

B. ALCOHOLISM AND ADDICTION

1045. Bourke, J.G.: Distillation by Early American Indians, *Amer Anthrop* 7:297–299, 1894.

1046. Horton, D.: The Functions of Alcohol in Primitive Societies; A Cross Cultural Study, *Quart J Stud Alcohol* 4:199–220, 1943.

1047. Honigmann, J.J., and Honigmann, I.: Drinking in an Indian-White Community, *Quart J Stud Alcohol* 5:575–619, 1945.

1048. Devereux, G.: The Function of Alcohol in Mohave Society, *Quart J Stud Alcohol* 9:207–251, 1948.

1049. Lemert, E.M.: *Alcoholism and Northwest Coast Indians*, U of Calif Publ in Culture and Society, vol 2 (No. 6) 1954, pp 304–406.

1050. Hawthorne, H.B.; Belshaw, C.S.; and Jamieson, S.M.: The Indians of British Columbia and Alcohol, *Alcohol Rev* 2:10–14, 1957.

1051. Lemert, E.M.: The Use of Alcohol in Three Salish Indian Tribes, *Quart J Stud Alcohol* 19:90–107, 1958.

1052. Baker, J.L.: Indians, Alcohol, and Homicide, *J Soc Ther* 5: 270–275, 1959.

1053. Bales, R.F.: *Cultural Differences in Rates of Alcoholism, Drinking, and Intoxication*, New Brunswick, NJ: Rutgers Center for Alcoholic Studies, 1959.

1054. Carpenter, E.S.: Alcohol in the Iroquois Dream Quest, *Amer J Psychiat* 116:148–151 (Aug) 1959.

1055. Clairmont, D.H.: *Notes on the Drinking Behavior of the Eskimos and Indians in the Aklavik Area, Canada*, Northern Coordination and Res Center, NCRC-62-4, 1962, p 13.

1056. Schaefer, O.: Alcohol Withdrawal Syndrome in a Newborn Infant of a Yukon Indian Mother, *Canad Med Ass J* 87:1333–1334 (Dec 22) 1962.

1057. Whittaker, J.O.: Alcohol and the Standing Rock Sioux Tribe, I: The Pattern of Drinking, *Quart J Stud Alcohol* 23:468–479, 1962.

1058. Whittaker, J.O.: Alcohol and the Standing Rock Sioux Tribe, II: Psychodynamic and Cultural Factors in Drinking, *Quart J Stud Alcohol* 24:80–90, 1963.

1059. Heath, D.B.: Prohibition and Post-Repeal Drinking Patterns Among the Navajo, *Quart J Stud Alcohol* 25:119–135, 1964.

1060. Pincock, T.A.: Alcoholism in Tuberculous Patients, *Canad Med Ass J* 91:851–854 (Oct) 1964.

1061. Hamer, J.H.: Acculturation Stress and the Functions of Alcohol Among the Forest Potawatomi, *Quart J Stud Alcohol* 26:285–302, 1965.

1062. Dozier, E.P.: Problem Drinking Among American Indians— The Role of Sociocultural Deprivation, *Quart J Stud Alcohol* 27:72–87, 1966.

1063. Mabry, D.E.: Pilot Study on Narcotic Control and Dispensing, abstracted, *Proc 1st Joint Meet of the Clin Soc and Commissioned Officers Ass USPHS*, Baltimore, Md (May) 1966, p 35.

1064. Curley, R.T.: Drinking Patterns of the Mescalero Apache, *Quart J Stud Alcohol* 28:116–131, 1967.

1065. Graves, T.D.: Acculturation Access and Alcoholism in Tri-Ethnic Community, *Amer Anthrop* 69:306–321, 1967.

1066. Kuttner, R.E., and Lorincz, A.B.: Alcoholism and Addiction in Urbanized Sioux Indians, *Ment Hyg* 51:530–542, 1967.

1067. Ferguson, F.N.: Navajo Drinking, *Hum Org* 27:159–167, 1968.

1068. Hayworth, D.D.: Alcoholism Pilot Study Program at US Public Health Service Hospital, Shiprock, New Mexico, abstracted, *Proc 3rd Joint Meet of the Clin Soc and Commissioned Officers Ass USPHS*, San Francisco, Calif (March) 1968, p 14.

1069. Savard, R.J.: Effects of Disulfiram Therapy on Relationships Within the Navajo Drinking Group, *Quart J Stud Alcohol* 29: 909–916, 1968.

1070. Sievers, M.L.: Cigarette and Alcohol Usage by Southwestern American Indians, *Amer J Public Health* 58:71–78 (Jan) 1968.

1071. Vall-Spinosa, A.: Antabuse Treatment of Alcoholism in Navajo and Hopi Indians, abstracted, *Proc 3rd Joint Meet of the Clin Soc and Commissioned Officers Ass USPHS*, San Francisco, Calif (March) 1968, p 23.

1072. Winkler, A.M.: Drinking on the American Frontier, *Quart J Study Alcohol* 29:413–445, 1968.

1073. *Alcoholism: A High Priority Health Problem*, US Public Health Serv, Health Serv and Mental Health Administration, Indian Health Serv (Dec) 1969.

1074. Henk, M.L.: Treatment Programs for the Navajo Alcoholic, abstracted, *Proc 4th Joint Meet of the Clin Soc and Commissioned Officers Ass USPHS*, Boston (June) 1969, p 48.

1075. *Indian Health Service: Preliminary Report of the Indian Health Service Task Force on Alcoholism*, US Public Health Serv, Health Serv and Mental Health Administration, Indian Health Serv (Jan) 1969.

C. SUICIDE

1076. Wyman, L., and Thorne, B.: Navajo Suicide, *Amer Anthrop* 47:278–288, 1945.

1077. Devereux, G.: *Mohave Ethnopsychiatry and Suicide: The Psychiatric Knowledge and the Psychic Disturbances of an Indian Tribe*, Smithsonian Inst, Bur of Amer Ethnology, Bull 175, 1961, p 586.

1078. Levy, J.E.: Navajo Suicide, *Hum Org* 24:308–318, 1965.

1079. Miller, S.I.: Suicide and Suicide Attempt Patterns Among the Navajo Indians, abstracted, *Proc 4th Joint Meet of the Clin Soc and Commissioned Officers Ass USPHS*, Boston (June) 1969, p 53.

D. PSYCHOTIC AND PSYCHONEUROTIC DISORDERS

1080. Hammer, H.R.: Insanity Among the Indians, *Proc Amer Med Psychol Ass* 19:453–462, 1912.

1081. Hammer, H.R.: Insanity Among the Indians, *Amer J Insanity* 69:615–623, 1913.

1082. Perkins, A.E.: Psychoses of the American Indians Admitted to Gowanda State Hospital, *Psychoanal Quart* 1:335–343, 1927.

1083. Pfister, O.: Instinctive Psychoanalysis Among the Navajos,

Imago 18:81–109, 1932; and *J Nerv Ment Dis* 76:234–254, 1932.

1084. Opler, M.E.: Points of Comparison and Contrast Between Treatment of Functional Disorders by Apache Shamans and Modern Psychiatric Practice, *Amer J Psychiat* 92:1371–1387, 1936.

1085. Landes, R.: The Abnormal Among the Ojibwa Indians, *J Abnorm Soc Psychol* 33:14–33, 1938.

1086. Devereux, G.: Primitive Psychiatry (Among Mohave Indians), *Bull Hist Med* 8:1194–1213, 1940.

1087. Leighton, A.H., and Leighton, D.C.: Elements of Psychotherapy in Navajo Religion, *Psychiatry* 4:515–523, 1941.

1088. Joseph, A.: Physician and Patient; Some Aspects of Interpersonal Relations Between Physicians and Patients, with Special Regard to the Relationship of White Physicians and Indian Patients, *Appl Anthrop* 1:1–6, 1941–1942.

1089. Devereux, G.: Primitive Psychiatry, Funeral Suicide, and Mohave Social Structure, *Bull Hist Med* 11:522–542, 1942.

1090. Leighton, A.H., and Leighton, D.C.: Some Types of Uneasiness and Fear in a Navajo Indian Community, *Amer Anthrop* 44:194–209, 1942.

1091. Bromberg, W., and Tranter, C.L.: Peyote Intoxication; Psychologic Aspects of Peyote Rite, *J Nerv Ment Dis* 97:518–527, 1943.

1092. Fischer, S.: Influence of Indian and Negro Blood on Manic-Depressive Psychoses, *J Nerv Ment Dis* 97:409–420, 1943.

1093. LaBarre, W.: Primitive Psychotherapy in Native American Cultures: Peyotism and Confession, *J Abnorm Soc Psychol* 42:294–309, 1947.

1094. Devereux, G.: Three Technical Problems in the Psychotherapy of Plains Indian Patients, *Amer J Psychother* 5:411–423 (July) 1951.

1095. Elmendorf, W.W.: "Soul Loss Illness in Western North America," in *International Congress of Americanists (29th), New York, 1949, Selected Papers*, vol 3: *Indian Tribes of Aboriginal America*, Chicago, 1952, pp 104–114.

1096. Anderson, C.M.: Psychiatrist Gives Medical Analysis of First 600 Cases Seen by Alaska Department of Health Mental Health Team, *Alaska's Health* 12:2–4 (Oct) 1955.

1097. Wallace, A.F.: Cultural Determinants of Response to Hallucinatory Experiment, *Arch Gen Psychiat* 1:58–69 (July) 1959.
1098. Slobodin, R.: Some Social Functions of Kutchin Anxiety, *Amer Anthrop* 62:122–133 (Feb) 1960.
1099. Nelson, L.G., et al: Screening for Emotionally Disturbed Students in an Indian Boarding School: Experience with the Cornell Medical Index Health Questionnaire, *Amer J Psychiat* 120:1155–1159 (June) 1964.
1100. Krush, T.P., et al: Some Thought on the Formation of Personality Disorder: Study of an American Indian Boarding School Population, *Amer J Psychiat* 122:868–876 (Feb) 1966.
1101. Stage, T.B., and Keast, T.J.: A Psychiatric Service for Plains Indians, *Hosp Community Psychiat* 17:74–76, 1966.
1102. Miles, J.E.: The Psychiatric Aspects of the Traditional Medicine of the British Columbia Coast Indian, *Canad Psychiat Ass J* 12:429–431 (Aug) 1967.
1103. Robertson, G.G., et al: Psychiatric Consultation on Two Indian Reservations, *Hosp Community Psychiat* 20:186–190 (Jan) 1969.

E. STUTTERING

1104. Johnson, W.: Indians Have No Word for It: Stuttering in Adults, *Quart J Speech* 30:456–465, 1944.
1105. Johnson, W.: Indians Have No Word for It: Stuttering in Children, *Quart J Speech* 30:330–337, 1944.
1106. Snidecor, J.C.: Why the Indian Does Not Stutter, *Quart J Speech* 33:493–495, 1947.
1107. Lemert, E.M.: Some Indians Who Stutter, *J Speech Hearing Dis* 18:168–174 (June) 1953.
1108. Stewart, J.L.: The Problem of Stuttering in Certain North American Indian Societies, *J Speech Hearing Dis* 25 (suppl 6):1–87 (April) 1960.

F. OTHER

1109. Shufeldt, R.W.: Modesty Among the North American Indians, *Alienist & Neurologist* 36:341–348, 1915.

1110. Walsh, J.J.: Mind and Body, *Ohio State Med J* 25:621–626, 1929.

1111. Telford, C.W.: Test Performance of Full and Mixed-Blood North Dakota Indians, *J Comp Psychol* 14:123–145, 1932.

1112. Devereux, G.: Institutionalized Homosexuality of Mohave Indians, *Hum Biol* 9:498–527, 1937.

1113. Devereux, G.: Social and Cultural Implications of Incest Among Mohave Indians, *Psychoanal Quart* 8:510–533, 1939.

1114. Devereux, G., and Loeb, E.M.: Apache Criminality, *J Crim Psychopath* 4:424–430, 1943.

1115. Arthur, G.: Experience in Examining a Twelfth-Grade Group with the Multiphasic Personality Inventory, *Ment Hyg* 28: 243–250, 1944.

1116. Havighurst, R.J.: *American Indian and White Children: A Sociopsychological Investigation*, Chicago: U of Chicago Press, 1955.

1117. Lemert, E.M., and Roseberg, J.: *The Administration of Justice to Minority Groups in Los Angeles County*, U of Calif Publ in Culture and Society, vol 2 (No. 1) 1955, pp 303–406.

1118. Klopper, B., and Boyer, L.B.: Notes on the Personality Structure of a North American Indian Shaman: Rorschach Interpretation, *J Project Techn* 25:170–178 (June) 1961.

1119. Carney, R.E., and Trowbridge, N.: Intelligence Test Performance of Indian Children as a Function of Type of Test and Age, *Percept Motor Skills* 14:511–514 (June) 1962.

1120. Boyer, L.B.: Comparison of the Shamans and Pseudoshamans of the Apaches of the Mescalero Indian Reservation: A Rorschach Study, *J Project Techn* 28:173–180, 1964.

1121. Stewart, O.: Questions Regarding American Indian Criminality, *Hum Org* 23:61–66, 1964.

1122. Kunce, J.; Rankin, L.S.; and Clement, E.: Maze Performance and Personal, Social, and Economic Adjustment of Alaskan Natives, *J Soc Psychol* 73:37–45 (Oct) 1967.

1123. Foster, A.: The Use of Psychological Testing in Rehabilitation Planning for Alaskan Native People, *Aust Psychologist* 4:146–152, 1969.

1124. Kern, M.: Uses of Clinical Hypnosis in the Setting of the Small Indian Health Service Health Station, abstracted, *Proc*

4th Joint Meet of the Clin Soc and Commissioned Officers Ass USPHS, Boston (June) 1969, p 40.

1125. Wolman, C.: Group Therapy in Two Languages, English and Navajo, abstracted, *Proc 4th Joint Meet of the Clin Soc and Commissioned Officers Ass USPHS*, Boston (June) 1969, p 21.

VIII. PREGNANCY, CHILDBIRTH, AND GYNECOLOGICAL CONDITIONS

1126. McClellan, E.: Obstetric Procedure Among Certain of the Aborigines of North America, *Proc Kentucky Med Soc*, 1873, pp 88–100.

1127. Bissell, G.P.: Description of Proceedings of the Clalam Squaws of Puget Sound, in Some Cases of Difficulty in Accouchement, *Calif Med J* 10:227, 1889.

1128. Holder, A.B.: The Age of Puberty of Indian Girls, *Amer J Obstet* 23:1074, 1890.

1129. Treon, F.: Obstetrics Among the Sioux Indian Women, *Cincinnati Lancet–Clinic* ns 24:12–14, 1890.

1130. Currier: A Study Relative to the Functions of Reproduction Apparatus in American Indian Women, *Trans Amer Gynec Soc* 16:264–294, 1891; and *Med News* 59:390–393, 1891.

1131. Barker, W.T.: Concerning American Indian Womanhood; An Ethnological Study, *Ann Gynaec & Paediat* 5:330–341, 1891–1892.

1132. Holder, A.B.: Gynecic Notes Taken Among the American Indians, *Amer J Obstet* 25:752, 1892; and 26:41, 1892.

1133. Simpson, J.K.: Midwifery Among the Alaskan Indians, *Occid Med Times* 6:61, 1892.

1134. Godfrey, G.C.M.: The Indian Woman in Labor, *Med Rec* 46:690, 1894.

1135. Grinnell, G.B.: Childbirth Among the Blackfeet, *Amer Anthrop* 9:285, 1896.

1136. King, J.C.: Obstetrics Among Aborigines, *Codex Med* 3:128–

133, 1896–1897; and *Southern Calif Practitioner* 12:41–45, 1897.

1137. Aberle, S.B.D.: Relation of Childbirth to Maternal Age and the Interval Between Births Among the Pueblo Indians, abstracted, *Eugen News* 13:100, 1928.

1138. Aberle, S.B.D.: Frequency of Pregnancies and Birth Interval Among Pueblo Indians, *Amer J Phys Anthrop* 16:63–80, 1931.

1139. Gilmore, M.R.: Notes on Gynecology and Obstetrics of the Arikara Tribe of Indians, *Papers Michigan Acad Sci Arts Letters* 14:71–81, 1931.

1140. Hrdlička, A.: Fecundity in the Sioux Women, *Amer J Phys Anthrop* 16:81–90, 1931.

1141. Sterling, E.B.: Maternal, Fetal, and Neonatal Mortality Among 1,815 Hospitalized Indians, *Public Health Rep* 48: 522–535, 1933; and *Amer J Phys Anthrop* 18:491–493, 1934.

1142. Aberle, S.B.D.: Maternal Mortality Among Pueblos, *Amer J Phys Anthrop* 18:431–435, 1934.

1143. Wissler, C.: Excess of Females Among the Cree Indians, *Proc Natl Acad Sci USA* 22:151–153, 1936.

1144. Rothrock, J.L.: Pregnancy and Childbirth Among North American Indians, *Minnesota Med* 22:750–756, 1939.

1145. Devereux, G.: Mohave Beliefs Concerning Twins, *Amer Anthrop* 43:573–592, 1941.

1146. Devereux, G.: Mohave Pregnancy, *Acta Americana* 6:89–116, 1948.

1147. McCammon, C.S.: A Study of Four Hundred Seventy-five Pregnancies in American Indian Woman, *Amer J Obstet* 61: 1159–1166 (May) 1951.

1148. Bailey, F.L.: *Some Sex Beliefs and Practices in a Navajo Community*, Cambridge, Mass: Peabody Mus of Amer Archeology and Ethnology Papers, 1955.

1149. Devereux, G.: *A Study of Abortion in Primitive Societies; A Typographical, Distributional, and Dynamic Analysis of the Prevention of Birth in 400 Preindustrial Societies*, New York: Julian Press, 1955.

1150. Thomas, G.W.: Pregnancy and Tuberculosis, *Canad Med Ass J* 81:710–714 (Nov) 1959.

1151. Langford, H.G., et al: Epidemiological Studies of Toxemia of Pregnancy and Hypertension, abstracted, *Circulation* 30 (suppl 3, pt 3):110 (Oct) 1964.

1152. Carpenter, C.W., and Bryans, B.: Maternal Mortality in British Columbia, *Canad Med Ass J* 92:168–169 (Jan) 1965.

1153. Loughlin, B.W.: Pregnancy in the Navajo Culture, *Nurs Outlook* 13:55–58 (March) 1965.

1154. Tyler, C.W., Jr., and Saeger, A.L., Jr.: Maternal Health in Non-Reservation American Indians, abstracted, *Proc 2nd Joint Meet of the Clin Soc and Commissioned Officers Ass USPHS*, Atlanta, Ga (May) 1967, p 1.

1155. Wallach, E.E.; Beer, A.E.; and Garcia, C.: Patient Acceptance of Oral Contraceptives, *Amer J Obstet Gynec* 97:984–991 (April) 1967.

1156. Adams, M.S.; MacLean, C.J.; and Niswander, J.D.: Discrimination Between Deviant and Ordinary Low Birth Weight: American Indian Infants, *Growth* 32:153–159, 1968.

1157. Adams, M.S., and Niswander, J.D.: Birth Weight of North American Indians, *Hum Biol* 40:226–234 (May) 1968.

1158. Leopardi, E.A.; Berg, L.E.; and Pournelle, A.T.: Indian Maternal-Infant Record Study, abstracted, *Proc 3rd Joint Meet of the Clin Soc and Commissioned Officers Ass USPHS*, San Francisco, Calif (March) 1968, p 73.

1159. Thomas, W.D.S.: Maternal Mortality in Native British Columbia Indians, a High Risk Group, *Canad Med Ass J* 99:64–67 (July) 1968.

1160. Holmes, R.H.: A Study of Obstetric Problems in an Indian Population, abstracted, *Proc 4th Joint Meet of the Clin Soc and Commissioned Officers Ass USPHS* Boston (June) 1969, p 60.

IX. CONGENITAL MALFORMATIONS

A. INBORN ERRORS OF METABOLISM

1161. Benedict, R.: "Why There Are Albinos," in *Zuni Mythology*, vol 2, New York: Columbia U Press, 1935, pp 207–210.

1162. Scott, E.M., and Hoskins, D.D.: Congenital Methemoglobinemia in Alaskan Indians and Eskimos, abstracted, *Sci in
Alaska*, Proc 7th Alaskan Sci Conf (1956), AAAS, Alaska Div,
pp 103–104.

1163. Scott, E.M., and Hoskins, D.D.: Hereditary Methemoglobinemia in Alaskan Eskimos and Indians, *Blood* 13:795–802
(Aug) 1958.

1164. Allison, A.C.; Blumberg, B.S.; and Gortler, S.M.: Urinary
Excretion of Beta-isobutyric Acid in Eskimo and Indian
Populations of Alaska, *Nature* 183:118–119, 1959.

1165. Scott, E.M.: A Test for the Enzymatic Deficiency of Hereditary Methemoglobinemia, *Alaska Med* 1:75–77, 1959.

1166. Scott, E.M.: The Relation of Diaphorase of Human Eryth-
rocytes to Inheritance of Methemoglobinemia, *J Clin Invest*
39:1176–1179 (July) 1960.

1167. Woolf, C.M., and Grant, R.B.: Albinism Among the Hopi
Indians in Arizona, *Amer J Hum Genet* 14:391–400 (Dec)
1962.

1168. Balsamo, P.; Hardy, E.R.; and Scott, E.M.: Hereditary Methemoglobinemia Due to Diaphorase Deficiency in Navajo
Indians, *J Pediat* 65:928–930 (Dec) 1964.

1169. Jones, J.A.: Rio Grande Pueblo Albinism, *Amer J Phys Anthrop* 22:265–270 (Sept) 1964.

1170. Woolf, C.M.: Albinism Among Indians in Arizona and New
Mexico, *Amer J Hum Genet* 17:23–35 (Jan) 1965.

1171. O'Brien, W.M.; Burch, T.A.; and Bunim, J.J.: Genetics of
Hyperuricaemia in Blackfeet and Pima Indians, *Ann Rheum
Dis* 24:117–119 (March) 1966.

1172. Bennett, P.H., and Burch, T.A.: "Serum Uric Acid and Gout
in Blackfeet and Pima Indians," in *Population Studies of
Rheumatic Diseases*, New York: Excerpta Med Foundation,
1967, p 359.

1173. Perry, T.L., and Finch, C.A.: Pentosuria in a North American
Indian, *Nature* 216:1027–1028 (Dec) 1967.

1174. Wagner, M.G., and Littman, B.: Phenylketonuria in the American Indians, *Pediatrics* 39:108–110 (Jan) 1967.

1175. Perry, T.L., et al: Hyperprolinaemia in Two Successive Generations of a North American Indian Family, *Ann Hum Genet* 31:404–407 (July) 1968.

1176. Woolf, C.M., et al: Hopi Indians, Inbreeding and Albinism, *Science* 164:30–37 (April 4) 1969.

B. OTHER

1177. Garth, T.R.: The Incidence of Color Blindness Among Races, *Science* 77:333–334, 1933.

1178. Hill, W.W.: The Status of the Hermaphrodite and Transvestite in Navaho Culture, *Amer Anthrop* ns 37:273–279, 1935.

1179. Bleyer, A.: Mongolism in a North American Indian, *J Missouri Med Ass* 33:13–14, 1936.

1180. Sirkin, J.: Mongolism Occurring in Indians, 3 Cases, *New York J Med* 37:167–168, 1937.

1181. Corrigan, C., and Sega, S.: The Incidence of Congenital Dislocation of the Hip at Island Lake, Manitoba, *Canad Med Ass J* 62:535–540 (June) 1950.

1182. Kraus, B.S.: Carabelli's Anomaly of Maxillary Molar Teeth; Observations on Mexicans and Papago Indians and Interpretation of Inheritance, *Amer J Hum Genet* 3:348–355 (Dec) 1951.

1183. Stewart, T.D.: The Age Incidence of Neural-Arch Defects in Alaskan Natives, Considered from the Standpoint of Etiology, *J Bone Joint Surg* [*Amer*] 35-A:937–950 (Oct) 1953.

1184. Stewart, T.D.: Examination of the Possibility that Certain Skeletal Characters Predispose to Defects in the Lumbar Neural Arches, *Clin Orthop* 8:44–60, 1956.

1185. Kraus, B.S., and Schwartzmann, J.R.: Congenital Dislocation of the Hip Among the Fort Apache Indians, abstracted, *J Bone Joint Surg* [*Amer*] 39-A:448–449 (April) 1957.

1186. Tretsven, V.E.: Incidence of Cleft Lip and Palate in Montana Indians, *J Speech Hearing Dis* 28:52–57 (Feb) 1963.

1187. Miller, J.R.: "The Use of Registries and Vital Statistics in the Study of Congenital Malformations," in *2nd Internatl Conf on Congen Malform*, New York: Internatl Med Congress, 1964, pp 334–340.

1188. Niswander, J.D., and Adams, M.S.: *American Indian Congenital Malformation Study; Summary of Newborn Record—July 1, 1964–June 30, 1965,* US Public Health Serv, Natl Inst Dent Res and Div of Indian Health, 1965.

1189. Rabin, D.L., et al: Untreated Congenital Hip Disease, *Amer J Public Health* 55 (suppl to Feb):1–44, 1965.

1190. Woolf, C.M.; Dolowitz, D.A.; and Aldous, H.E.: Congenital Deafness and Piebaldness in Two American Indian Brothers, *Arch Otolaryng* 82:244–250 (Sept) 1965.

1191. Niswander, J.D., and Adams, M.S.: *American Indian Congenital Malformation Study—Summary of Newborn Record —July 1, 1964–June 20, 1966,* US Public Health Serv, Natl Inst Dent Res and Div of Indian Health, 1966.

1192. Yost, G.: Two Cases of Anhidrotic Ectodermal Dysplasia in Indians of the Southwest, abstracted, *Proc 1st Joint Meet of the Clin Soc and Commissioned Officers Ass USPHS,* Baltimore, Md (May) 1966, p 7.

1193. Ballestero, R.J., and Goble, M.G.: Kartagener's Syndrome in an American Indian Girl, *Dis Chest* 51:227–228 (Feb) 1967.

1194. Curzon, J.A., and Curzon, M.E.: Congenital Dental Anomalies in a Group of British Columbia Children, *J Canad Dent Ass* 33:554–558 (Oct) 1967.

1195. Flynn, L.R.: Oculomandibulodyscephaly: Hallerman-Streiff Syndrome, abstracted, *Proc 2nd Joint Meet of the Clin Soc and Commissioned Officers Ass USPHS,* Atlanta, Ga (May) 1967, p 63.

1196. Niswander, J.D., and Adams, M.S.: Oral Clefts in the American Indian, *Public Health Rep* 82:807–812 (Sept) 1967.

1197. Adams, M.S., and Niswander, J.D.: Health of the American Indian, Congenital Defects, *Eugen Quart* 15:227–234, 1968.

1198. Harris, R.L., and Riley, H.D., Jr.: Cystic Fibrosis in the American Indian, *Pediatrics* 41:733–738 (April) 1968.

1199. Jaffe, B.: Congenital Aural Atresia in Navajo Indians, abstracted, *Proc 3rd Joint Meet of the Clin Soc and Commissioned Officers Ass USPHS,* San Francisco, Calif (March) 1968, p 10.

1200. Shapiro, B.L.: Bifid Uvula in Chippewa Indian Children, abstracted, *Internatl Ass Dent Res—Abstracts*, 1968, p 122 (Abstract 337).

1201. Comess, L.J.: Congenital Anomalies and Diabetes in the Pima Indians of Arizona, *Diabetes* 18:471–477 (July) 1969.

1202. Craniofacial Birth Defects Can Elude Recognition and Management, *JAMA* 208:2003 (June) 1969.

1203. Lowry, R.B., and Renwick, D.H.G.: Incidence of Cleft Lip and Palate in British Columbia Indians, *J Med Genet* 6:67–69 (Jan) 1969.

X. CHILD HEALTH AND DISEASES OF INFANCY OTHER THAN MALFORMATIONS

1204. Aberle, S.B.D.: Child Mortality Among Pueblo Indians, *Amer J Phys Anthrop* 16:339–349, 1937.

1205. Pijoan, M., and Elkin, C.A.: Secondary Anemia Due to Prolonged and Exclusive Milk Feeding Among Shoshone Indian Infants, *J Nutr* 27:67–75, 1944.

1206. Devereux, G.: Mohave Indian Infanticide, *Psychoanal Rev* 35:126–139, 1948.

1207. Hayman, C.R.: Chronic Disease Program for Children Expanded, *Alaska's Health* 13:1–2 (Feb) 1956.

1208. Hayman, C.R., and Kester, F.E.: A Study of Infant Mortality in Alaska, *Northwest Med* 56:819–823 (July) 1957.

1209. Study of Causes of Death of Alaska Infants, *Alaska's Health* 14:1–2 (April) 1957.

1210. Navajo Child Health Level Mirrors Tribe Future, *Public Health Rep* 73:250 (March) 1958.

1211. Lizotte, A.: Infantile Diarrhea and Gastroenteritis, Churchill, Manitoba, *Canad Serv Med J* 15:421–433 (July–Aug) 1959.

1212. Perking, G.B., and Church, G.M.: Report of Pediatric Evaluations of a Sample of Indian Children—Wind River Indian Reservation, 1957, *Amer J Public Health* 50:181–194 (Feb) 1960.

1213. Pasinsky, S.H.: Navaho Infancy and Childhood, *Psychiat Quart* 37:306–321 (April) 1963.

1214. Riley, H.D., Jr., et al: Report of the Committee on Indian Health: The Pediatrician and Indian Health, *Pediatrics* 36: 958–961 (Dec) 1965.

1215. Rosa, F., and Resnick, L.: Birth Weight and Perinatal Mortality in the American Indian, *Amer J Obstet Gynec* 91:972–976 (April) 1965.

1216. Riley, H.D., Jr.: Child Health Among Indians, *J Oklahoma Med Ass* 59:88–89, 1966.

1217. French, J.G.: Relationship of Morbidity to the Feeding Patterns of Navajo Children from Birth Through Twenty-four Months, *Amer J Clin Nutr* 20:375–385 (May) 1967.

1218. Graham-Cumming, G.: Hygiène Prénatale et Mortalité Infantile Chez les Indiens, *Infirm Canad* 9:34–35 (Sept) 1967.

1219. Graham-Cumming, G.: Infant Care in Canadian Indian Homes, *Canad J Public Health* 58:391–394 (Sept) 1967.

1220. Graham-Cumming, G.: Prenatal Care and Infant Mortality Among Canadian Indians, *Canad Nurse* 63:29–31 (Sept) 1967.

1221. Gurunanjappa, B.S.: Alaska Native Infant Health Problem, *Alaska Med* 9:88–93, 1967.

1222. McGee, M.D.: Six Years of Well Child Clinic Experience at the Phoenix Service Unit, abstracted, *Proc 2nd Joint Meet of the Clin Soc and Commissioned Officers Ass USPHS*, Atlanta, Ga (May) 1967, p 48.

1223. Newton, J.B.: Pneumonia in Indian and Eskimo Infants in Canada, *Canad Med Ass J* 96:1334–1335 (May) 1967.

1224. Brenneman, G.: Battered Child Syndrome, *Alaska Med* 10: 175–178, 1968.

1225. Infant Life and Infant Mortality, *Public Health Serv World* (April) 1968, pp 13–15.

XI. DISEASES OF THE INTEGUMENTARY SYSTEM

1226. Fox, H.: Diseases of the Skin in Oklahoma Indians, *Arch Derm Syph* 40:544–546, 1936.

1227. Everett, M.A., et al: Light-Sensitive Eruptions in American Indians, *Arch Derm* 83:243–248 (Feb) 1961.

1228. Farber, E.M.; Grauer, F.; and Zaruba, F.: Racial Incidence of Psoriasis, *Cesk Derm* 40:289–297, 1965.

1229. Birt, A.R.: Photodermatitis in Indians of Manitoba, *Canad Med Ass J* 98:392–397 (Feb) 1968.

1230. Berger, L.S.: Lipidematous Alopecia in the Navajo, abstracted, *Proc 4th Joint Meet of the Clin Soc and Commissioned Officers Ass USPHS,* Boston (June) 1969, p 13.

XII. DISEASES OF THE MUSCULOSKELETAL SYSTEM

1231. Dunham, C.L., and Montross, H.E.: Atrophic Arthritis Among Pima Indians of Arizona, *Amer J Med Sci* 193:229–233, 1937.

1232. Gray, C.G.: Some Orthopaedic Problems in Indians and Eskimos, *Canad J Occup Ther* 27:45–50 (June) 1960.

1233. Burch, T.A.; O'Brien, W.M.; and Bunim, J.J.: Occurrence of Rheumatoid Arthritis and Rheumatoid Factor in Families of Blackfeet Indians, abstracted, *Arthritis Rheum* 5:640 (Dec) 1962.

1234. Robinson, H.S., and Gofton, J.P.: An Epidemiological Study of the Prevalence of Arthritis in the Haida Indians, abstracted, *Arthritis Rheum* 5:657 (Dec) 1962.

1235. Burch, T.A.: A Comparison of the Prevalence of Rheumatoid Arthritis (RA) and Rheumatoid Factor (RF) in Indian Tribes Living in Montana Mountains and in Arizona Desert, abstracted, *Arthritis Rheum* 6:765 (Dec) 1963.

1236. O'Brien, W.M.; Burch, T.A.; and Bunim, J.J.: A Genetic Analysis of the Occurrence of Rheumatoid Factor (RF) and Rheumatoid Arthritis (RA) in 485 Matings and 1633 Sibling Pairs in Pima and Blackfeet Indians, abstracted, *Arthritis Rheum* 6:785–786 (Dec) 1963.

1237. Price, G.E., et al: An Outbreak of "Infectious" Polyarthritis in a Haida Indian Family, *Arthritis Rheum* 6:633–638 (Oct) 1963.

1238. Robinson, H.S.; Gofton, J.P.; and Price, G.E.: A Study of Rheumatic Disease in a Canadian Indian Population, *Ann Rheum Dis* 22:232–236 (July) 1963.

1239. Robinson, H.S.; Gofton, J.P.; and Price, G.E.: Marie-Strumpell Spondylitis in the Haida Indians, abstracted, *Arthritis Rheum* 6:293 (June) 1963.

1240. Bunim, J.J.; Burch, T.A.; and O'Brien, W.M: Influence of Genetic and Environmental Factors on Occurrence of Rheumatoid Arthritis and Rheumatoid Factor in American Indians, *Bull Rheum Dis* 15:349–350 (Sept) 1964.

1241. Burch, T.A.; O'Brien, W.M.; and Bunim, J.J.: Family and Genetic Studies of Rheumatoid Arthritis and Rheumatoid Factor in Blackfeet Indians, *Amer J Public Health* 54:1184–1190 (Aug) 1964.

1242. Burch, T.A., et al: Prevalencia de Artritis Reumatoidea y Factor Reumatoideo en Indios Americanos, *Rev Med Chile* 92:183–186, 1964.

1243. Gofton, J.P.; Robinson, H.S.; and Price, G.E.: A Study of Rheumatic Disease in a Canadian Indian Population, II: Rheumatoid Arthritis in the Haida Indians, *Ann Rheum Dis* 23:364–371 (Sept) 1964.

1244. Morris, J.W.: Skeletal Fluorosis Among Indians of the American Southwest, *Amer J Roentgen* 94:608–615 (July) 1965.

1245. Burch, T.A.: Epidemiological Studies on Rheumatic Diseases, *Milit Med* 131:507–512, 1966.

1246. Gofton, J.P.; Robinson, H.S.; and Truemen, G.E.: Ankylosing Spondylitis in a Canadian Indian Population, *Ann Rheum Dis* 25:525–527 (Nov) 1966.

1247. Gofton, J.P., et al: Sacroileitis in Eight Populations, *Ann Rheum Dis* 25:528–533 (Nov) 1966.

1248. Lawrence, J.S., et al: Geographical Studies on Rheumatoid Arthritis, *Ann Rheum Dis* 25:425–431 (Sept) 1966.

1249. Bennett, P.H., and Burch, T.A.: "The Epidemiologic Diagnosis of Ankylosing Spondylitis," in Bennett, P.H., and Wood, P.H.N. (eds.): *Population Studies of the Rheumatic Diseases*, New York: Excerpta Med Foundation, 1967, p 305.

1250. Bennett, P.H., and Burch, T.A.: "The Genetics of Rheumatoid Arthritis," in Bennett, P.H., and Wood, P.H.N. (eds.): *Popu-*

lation Studies of the Rheumatic Diseases, New York: Excerpta Med Foundation, 1967, p 136.

1251. Bennett, P.H., and Burch, T.A.: "Osteoarthrosis in the Blackfeet and Pima Indians," in Bennett, P.H., and Wood, P.H.N. (eds.): *Population Studies of the Rheumatic Diseases,* New York: Excerpta Med Foundation, 1967, p 407.

1252. Gofton, J.P., et al: "Sacroileitis in Eight Populations," in Bennett, P.H., and Wood, P.H.N. (eds.): *Population Studies of the Rheumatic Diseases,* New York: Excerpta Med Foundation, 1967, p 293.

1253. O'Brien, W.M., et al: A Genetic Study of Rheumatoid Arthritis and Rheumatoid Factor in Blackfeet and Pima Indians, *Arthritis Rheum* 10:163–179 (June) 1967.

1254. Senter, R.G.; Bennett, P.H.; and Burch, T.A.: Hyperostotic Spondylosis Among the Gila River Indians, abstracted, *Proc 3rd Joint Meet of the Clin Soc and Commissioned Officers Ass USPHS,* San Francisco, Calif (March) 1968, p 11.

1255. Hill, R.H., et al: Juvenile Rheumatoid Arthritis: A Medical and Social Profile of Non-Indian and Indian Children, *Canad Med Ass J* 100:458–464 (March 8) 1969.

XIII. DISEASES OF THE RESPIRATORY SYSTEM (CHRONIC)

1256. *(Eleventh) Annual Report of the Bureau of American Ethnology, 1889–1890,* Smithsonian Inst, Bur of Amer Ethnology, 1894, p 187.

1257. Herxheimer, H.: Asthma in American Indians, *N Eng J Med* 270:1128–1129 (May) 1964.

1258. Brown, G.W.: Report on Empyema Among Alaska Native Children: A Study of 22 Cases from the Alaska Native Medical Center, Anchorage, Alaska, *Alaska Med* 8:71–76, 1966.

1259. Wilson, J.F.; Cohen, J.; and Decker, A.: An Incidence Study of Bronchiectasis by Random Bronchography, abstracted, *Proc 1st Joint Meet of the Clin Soc and Commissioned Officers Ass USPHS,* Baltimore, Md (May) 1966, p 59.

1260. Fleshman, J.K.; Wilson, J.F.; and Cohen, J.J.: Bronchiectasis in Alaskan Native Children, *Arch Environ Health* 17:517–524 (Oct) 1968.

1261. Geller, A.: Desquamative Interstitial Pneumonia, abstracted, *Proc 3rd Joint Meet of the Clin Soc and Commissioned Officers Ass USPHS,* San Francisco, Calif (March) 1968, p 46.

1262. Sparger, C.F.: Foreign Bodies in the Tracheobronchial Tree and Esophagus, *Rocky Mountain Med J* 65:47–52 (April) 1968.

XIV. DISEASES OF THE CARDIOVASCULAR SYSTEM

1263. Paul, J.R., and Dixon, G.L.: Climate and Rheumatic Heart Disease; Survey Among American Indian School Children in Northern and Southern Localities, *JAMA* 108:2096–2100, 1937.

1264. Cohen, B.M.: Arterial Hypertension Among Indians of the Southwestern United States, *Amer J Med Sci* 225:505–513 (May) 1953.

1265. Gilbert, J: Absence of Coronary Thrombosis in Navajo Indians, *Calif Med* 82:114–115 (Feb) 1955.

1266. Noble, T.B.: Metabolic Aspects of Atherosclerosis (As Seen in the Three Aged Hopi Indians), *J Indiana Med Ass* 48:883–884, 1955.

1267. Page, I.H.; Lewis, L.A.; and Gilbert, J.: Plasma Lipids and Proteins and Their Relationship to Coronary Disease Among Navajo Indians, *Circulation* 13:675–679 (May) 1956.

1268. *Heart Disease Among Indians in the United States, 1955,* US Public Health Serv, Div of Indian Health, 1957.

1269. Smith, R.L.: Cardiovascular-Renal and Diabetes Deaths Among the Navajos, *Public Health Rep* 72:33–38 (Jan) 1957.

1270. Leo, T.F.; Kelly, J.J., Jr.; and Eder, H.A.: Cardiovascular Survey in a Population of Arizona Indians, abstracted, *Circulation* 18:748 (Oct) 1958.

1271. Abraham, S., and Miller, D.C.: Serum Cholesterol Levels in American Indians, *Public Health Rep* 74:392–398 (May) 1959.

1272. Straus, R.; Gilbert, J.; and Wurm, M.: Biochemical Studies in Full-Blooded Navajo Indians, *Circulation* 19:420–423 (March) 1959.

1273. Streeper, R.B., et al: An Electrocardiographic and Autopsy Study of Coronary Heart Disease in the Navajo, *Dis Chest* 38:305–312 (Sept) 1960.

1274. Kositchek, R.J.; Wurm, M.; and Straus, R.: Biochemical Studies in Full-Blooded Navajo Indians, II: Lipids and Lipoproteins, *Circulation* 23:219–224 (Feb) 1961.

1275. Clifford, N.J., et al: Coronary Heart Disease and Hypertension in the White Mountain Apache Tribe, *Circulation* 28:926–931 (Nov) 1963.

1276. Fulmer, H.S.: Coronary Heart Disease Among the Navajo Indians, *Ann Intern Med* 59:740–764 (Nov) 1963.

1277. Maynard, J.E.; Hammes, L.M.; and Kester, F.E.: Mortality Due to Heart Disease Among Alaskan Natives, 1955–1965, *Public Health Rep* 82:714–720 (Aug) 1967.

1278. Sievers, M.L.: Myocardial Infarction Among Southwestern American Indians, *Ann Intern Med* 67:807–817 (Oct) 1967.

1279. Bennett, P.H.; Burch, T.A.; and Liebow, I.M.: Epidemiologic Study of Coronary Heart Disease: Its Relationships to Diabetes Mellitus and Other Variables, abstracted, *Proc 3rd Joint Meet of the Clin Soc and Commissioned Officers Ass USPHS*, San Francisco, Calif (March) 1968, p 60.

1280. Sievers, M.L.: Serum Cholesterol Levels in Southwestern American Indians, *J Chron Dis* 21:107–115 (May) 1968.

XV. DISEASES OF THE HEMATOPOIETIC SYSTEM INCLUDING HEMOGLOBINOPATHIES

1281. Prouty, M.: Familial Erythroblastic (Cooley's) Anemia in an Infant, *Amer J Dis Child* 79:99–104 (Jan) 1950.

1282. Millar, J.: Some Observations on Hemoglobin Levels of an Indian Population, *Canad Med Ass J* 67:414–417 (Nov) 1952.

1283. Porter, V.S.; Wright, R.E.; and Scott, E.M.: "Anemia in

Western Alaska," in *Sci in Alaska*, Proc 4th Alaskan Sci Conf (1953), AAAS, Alaska Div, 1956, pp 217–219.

1284. Pollitzer, W.S., et al: Hemoglobin Patterns in American Indians, *Science* 129:216 (Jan) 1959.

1285. Scott, E.M., et al: Lack of Abnormal Hemoglobins in Alaskan Eskimos, Indians, and Aleuts, *Science* 129:719–720 (March) 1959.

1286. Hampton, J.E.: Pernicious Anemia in American Indians, *J Oklahoma Med Ass* 53:503–509 (July) 1960.

1287. Painter, S.L., and Elett, R.: Hemophilia (AHG Deficiency) and Factor VII (Stable Factor) Deficiency in the American Indians: Report of Four Cases, *Rocky Mountain Med J* 57:65–68 (Jan) 1960.

1288. Githens, J.H.: Prevalence of Abnormal Hemoglobins in American Indian Children: Survey in the Rocky Mountain Area, *J Lab Clin Med* 57:755–758 (May) 1961.

1289. Schneider, R.G., et al: Hemoglobin G-Coushatta: A New Variant in an American Indian Family, *Science* 143:697–698 (Feb) 1964.

1290. Brown, C.V.; Brown, G.W.; and Bonehill, B.: Relationship of Anemia to Infectious Illnesses on Kodiak Island, *Alaska Med* 9:93–95, 1967.

1291. Frederiksen, M.J., and McDonald, B.S.: Anemia in Navajo Indian Children, abstracted, *Proc 3rd Joint Meet of the Clin Soc and Commissioned Officers Ass USPHS*, San Francisco, Calif (March) 1968, p 47.

1292. Blackwell, R.O., et al: Hemoglobin Variant Found in Koreans, Chinese, and North American Indians: Alpha-2, Beta-2, 22 Glu-Ala, *Amer J Phys Anthrop* 30:389–391 (May) 1969.

XVI. DISEASES OF THE DIGESTIVE SYSTEM

A. GALLBLADDER DISEASE

1293. Lam, R.C.: Gallbladder Diseases Among the American Indians, *J Lancet* 74:305–309 (Aug) 1954.

1294. Hesse, F.G.: Incidence of Cholecystitis and Other Diseases Among Pima Indians of Southern Arizona, *JAMA* 170:1789–1790 (Aug) 1959.

1295. Sievers, M.L., and Marquis, J.R.: The Southwestern American Indians' Burden: Biliary Disease, *JAMA* 182:570 (Nov) 1962.

1296. Kravetz, R.E.: Etiology of Biliary Tract Disease in Southwestern American Indians, *Gastroenterology* 46:392–398 (April) 1964.

1297. Brown, J.E., and Christensen, C.: Biliary Tract Disease Among the Navajos, *JAMA* 202:1050–1052 (Dec) 1967.

1298. Comess, L.J.; Bennett, P.H.; and Burch, T.A.: Clinical Gallbladder Disease in Pima Indians, *N Eng J Med* 277:894–898 (Oct) 1967.

1299. Comess, L.J.; Burch, T.A.; and Bennett, P.H.: Prevalence of Gallbladder Disease Among the Pima Indians: Preliminary Report, abstracted, *Proc 2nd Joint Meet of the Clin Soc and Commissioned Officers Ass USPHS*, Atlanta, Ga (May) 1967, p 65.

1300. Burch, T.A.; Comess, L.J.; and Bennett, P.H.: "The Problem of Gallbladder Disease Among Pima Indians," in *Biomedical Challenges Presented by the American Indian*, WHO, Pan Amer Health Org, Publ 165, 1968, pp 82–88.

1301. Danielson, B.D.: Biliary Tract Disease in Navajo Indians, Letter to the Editor, *JAMA* 203:1073 (March 18) 1968.

1302. Sampliner, J.E., and O'Connell, D.J.: Biliary Surgery in the Southwestern American Indian, *Arch Surg* 96:1–3 (Jan) 1968.

B. OTHER

1303. Bebchuck, W.; Rogers, A.G.; and Downey, J.L.: Chronic Ulcerative Colitis in a North American Indian, *Gastroenterology* 40:138–140 (Jan) 1961.

1304. Sievers, M.L., and Marquis, J.R.: Duodenal Ulcer Among Southwestern American Indians, *Gastroenterology* 42:566–569 (May) 1962.

1305. Hislop, D.M.C.: A Case of Dublin-Johnson Syndrome in a North American Cree Indian with Suggestive Evidence of

Familial Occurrence, *Med Serv J Canada* 20:61–64 (Jan) 1964.

1306. Kuttner, R.E.: Serum Pepsinogen in Urbanized Sioux Indians, *J Natl Med Ass* 56:471 (Nov) 1964.

1307. Rogers, B.H.G., and Freimark, L.G.: Unusual Complications of Trichobezoar, *Amer J Dis Child* 110:215–217 (Aug) 1965.

1308. Sievers, M.L.: A Study of Achlorhydria Among Southwestern American Indians, *Amer J Gastroent* 45:99–108 (Feb) 1966.

1309. McGee, M.D., and Chabon, R.S.: Portal Hypertension in Childhood: Report of an Unusual Case and Subject Review, abstracted, *Proc 2nd Joint Meet of the Clin Soc and Commissioned Officers Ass USPHS*, Atlanta, Ga (May) 1967, p 74.

1310. Sparger, C.F.: Injury of the Upper Gastrointestinal Tract Due to Drinking "Battery Acid," *Virginia Med Mon* 95:679–682 (Nov) 1968.

1311. Kunitz, S.J., et al: Alcoholic Cirrhosis Among the Navajo, *Quart J Stud Alcohol* 30:672–685, 1969.

XVII. DISEASES OF THE ENDOCRINE SYSTEM

A. DIABETES MELLITUS

1312. Joslin, E.P.: The Universality of Diabetes, *JAMA* 115:2033–2038, 1940.

1313. Joslin, E.P., et al: *The History of Diabetes*, Philadelphia: Lea and Febiger, 1952, p 28.

1314. Cohen, B.M.: Diabetes Mellitus Among Indians of the American Southwest: Its Prevalence and Clinical Characteristics in a Hospitalized Population, *Ann Intern Med* 40:588–599 (March) 1954.

1315. Joslin, E.P., et al: *The History of Diabetes*, 10th ed, Philadelphia: Lea and Febiger, 1959, pp 41–44.

1316. Parks, J.H., and Waskow, E.: Diabetes Among the Pima Indians of Arizona, *Arizona Med* 18:99–106 (April) 1961.

1317. Drevets, C.C.: *Pilot Study of Diabetes Among Choctaw and Talihama*, Oklahoma City (Sept 6) 1962.

1318. Johnson, J.E., and McNutt, C.W.: Diabetes Mellitus in an American Indian Population Isolate, *Texas Rep Biol Med* 22:110 (Spring) 1964.

1319. Drevets, C.C.: Diabetes Mellitus in Choctaw Indians, *J Oklahoma Med Ass* 58:322–329, 1965.

1320. Miller, M., et al: Prevalence of Diabetes Mellitus in the American Indians: Results of Glucose Tolerance Tests in the Pima Indians of Arizona, abstracted, *Diabetes* 14:439 (July) 1965.

1321. Stein, J.H., et al: The High Prevalence of Abnormal Glucose Tolerance in the Cherokee Indians of North Carolina, *Arch Intern Med* 116:842–845 (Dec) 1965.

1322. Ede, M.C.: Diabetes and the Way of Life on an Indian Reservation, *Guy Hosp Rep* 115:455, 1966.

1323. White, W.D.: Diabetes in the Oklahoma Indian, abstracted, *Proc 1st Joint Meet of the Clin Soc and Commissioned Officers Ass USPHS*, Baltimore, Md (May) 1966, p 21.

1324. Genuth, S.M., et al: Hyperinsulinism in Obese Diabetic Pima Indians, *Metabolism* 16:1010–1015 (Nov) 1967.

1325. Henry, R.E.; Burch, T.A.; and Bennett, P.H.: Diabetes in the Cocopah Indians, abstracted, *Proc 2nd Joint Meet of the Clin Soc and Commissioned Officers Ass USPHS*, Atlanta, Ga (May) 1967, p 7.

1326. Prosnitz, L.R., and Mandell, G.L.: Diabetes Mellitus Among Navajo and Hopi Indians: The Lack of Vascular Complications, *Amer J Med Sci* 253:700–705 (June) 1967.

1327. Miller, M.; Bennett, P.H.; and Burch, T.A.: "Hyperglycemia in Pima Indians: A Preliminary Appraisal of Its Significance," in *Biomedical Challenges Presented by the American Indian*, WHO, Pan Amer Health Org, Publ 165, 1968, pp 89–103.

1328. Niswander, J.D.: "Some Special Medical Problems of Indian Populations—Discussion on Diabetes," in *Biomedical Challenges Presented by the American Indian*, WHO, Pan Amer Health Org, Publ 165, 1968, p 133.

1329. Rimoin, D.L., and Saiki, J.H.: Diabetes Mellitus Among the

Navajo, II: Plasma, Glucose, and Insulin Responses, *Arch Intern Med* 122:6–9 (July) 1968.

1330. Saiki, J.H., and Rimoin, D.L.: Diabetes Mellitus Among the Navajo, I: Clinical Features, *Arch Intern Med* 122:1–5 (July) 1968.

1331. Comess, L.J., et al: Congenital Anomalies and Diabetes in the Pima Indians of Arizona, *Diabetes* 18:471–477 (July) 1969.

1331A. Doeblin, T.D., et al: Diabetes and Hyperglycemia in Seneca Indians, *Hum Heredity* 19:613–627, 1969.

1332. Frohman, L.A.; Doeblin, T.D.; and Emerling, F.G.: Diabetes in the Seneca Indians, *Diabetes* 18:38–43 (Jan) 1969.

1333. Henry, R.E., et al: Diabetes in the Cocopah Indians, *Diabetes* 18:33–37 (Jan) 1969.

1334. Mouratoff, G.J.; Carroll, N.V.; and Scott, E.M.: Diabetes Mellitus in Athabaskan Indians in Alaska, *Diabetes* 18:29–32 (Jan) 1969.

1335. Petersen, K.: A Profile of Diabetes Mellitus Among the Indians of a Sioux Assiniboin Reservation, abstracted, *Proc 4th Joint Meet of the Clin Soc and Commissioned Officers Ass USPHS*, Boston (June) 1969, p 35.

1336. Rimoin, D.L.: Ethnic Variability in Glucose Tolerance and Insulin Secretion, *Arch Intern Med* 124:695–700 (Dec) 1969.

B. Other

1337. Rodahl, K., and Bang, G.: *Endemic Goiter in Alaska*, US Air Force, Arctic Aeromed Lab Techn, Note 56–59, 1956, p 8.

1338. Edwards, A.M., and Gray, G.C.: Observations on Juvenile Hypothyroidism in Native Races of Northern Canada, *Canad Med Ass J* 84:1116–1124 (May) 1961.

1339. Rodahl, K., and Bang, G.: Endemic Goiter in Alaska, *Arch Environ Health* 4:11–21, 1962.

1340. Monahan, G.F.: Addison's Disease: Three Cases Seen Among Indians and Eskimos of Hudson Bay, *Med Serv J Canada* 19:647–652 (Sept) 1963.

1341. Keefer, F.J.: Sheehan's Syndrome: A Case Report, *Alaska Med* 6:75–77, 1964.

1342. Osborne, M.D.: Endocrine Disturbances in Four Patients with Amenorrhea, abstracted, *Proc 1st Joint Meet of the Clin Soc and Commissioned Officers Ass USPHS*, Baltimore, Md (May) 1966, p 14.

1343. Saiki, J.H.: Severe Myxedema Following Inadvertent Removal of an Ectopic Thyroid Resembling a Thyroglossal Duct Cyst, *Lancet* 87:7–9 (Jan) 1967.

1344. Barzelatto, J., and Covarrubias, E.: "Study of Endemic Goiter in the American Indian," in *Biomedical Challenges Presented by the American Indian*, WHO, Pan Amer Health Org, Publ 165 (Sept) 1968, pp 124–132.

1345. Librik, L., et al: Thyrotoxicosis and Collagen-like Disease in Three Sisters of American Indian Extraction, *J Pediat* 76:64–68 (Jan) 1970.

XVIII. DISEASES OF THE UROGENITAL SYSTEM

1346. Westley, R., et al: Familial Nephritis in Southwestern Apache Indian Family, abstracted, *Proc 1st Joint Meet of the Clin Soc and Commissioned Officers Ass USPHS*, Baltimore, Md (May) 1966, p 20.

1347. Lobban, M.D.: Daily Rhythm of Renal Excretion in Arctic Dwelling Indians and Eskimos, *Quart J Exp Physiol* 52:401–410, 1967.

XIX. DISEASES OF THE NERVOUS SYSTEM

1348. Adams, G.S., and Kanner, L.: General Paralysis Among the North American Indians, *Amer J Psychol* 83:125–133, 1926.

1349. Adams, G.S., and Kanner, L.: General Paralysis Among North American Indians, *Arch Internatl Neurol* 1:168–170, 1927.

1350. Meehan, J.P.; Stoll, A.M.; and Hardy, J.D.: Cutaneous Pain Threshold in Native Alaskan Indians and Eskimos, *J Appl Physiol* 6:397–400 (Jan) 1954.

XX. DISEASES OF THE SENSE ORGANS

A. EYE

i. Phlyctenular Kerato-conjunctivitis

1351. Fritz, M.H., and Thygeson, P.: "Phlyctenular Kerato-conjunctivitis Among Alaskan Natives," in *Sci in Alaska*, Proc 1st Alaskan Sci Conf (1950), Natl Res Council Bull 122, 1951.

1352. Fritz, M.H., and Thygeson, P.: Public Health Problems in Alaska; Phlyctenular Kerato-conjunctivitis Among Alaskan Indians and Eskimos, *Public Health Rep* 66:934–939 (July) 1951.

1353. Fritz, M.H.; Thygeson, P.; and Durham, D.G.: Phlyctenular Kerato-conjunctivitis Among Alaskan Natives, *Amer J Ophthal* 34:177–184 (Feb) 1951.

1354. Thygeson, P.: The Etiology and Treatment of Phlyctenular Kerato-conjunctivitis, *Amer J Ophthal* 34:1217–1236 (Sept) 1951.

1355. Thygeson, P., and Fritz, M.H.: Cortisone in the Treatment of Phlyctenular Kerato-conjunctivitis, *Amer J Ophthal* 34:357–360 (March) 1951.

1356. Leer, R.H.: Phlyctenular Eye Disease in Alaska, abstracted, *Sci in Alaska*, Proc 7th Alaskan Sci Conf (1956), AAAS, Alaska Div, pp 99–100.

1357. Duggan, J.W., and Hatfield, R.E.: Phlyctenular Kerato-conjunctivitis, *Amer J Ophthal* 46:210–212 (Aug) 1958.

ii. Other

1358. Nichols, J.V.V.: A Survey of the Ophthalmic Status of the Cree Indians at Norway House, Manitoba, *Canad Med Ass J* 54:344–348 (April) 1946.

1359. Fritz, M.H.: Corneal Opacities Among Alaska Natives, *Alaska's Health* 5:3–7 (Dec) 1947.

1360. Kronenberg, B.: Survey of Ocular Conditions Among the Navajo-Hopi Indians, *Sightsav Rev* 27:7–11, 1957.

1361. Belloc, N.B.; Fowler, D.M.; and Simmons, W.H.: Causes of Blindness in California, *Sightsav Rev* 27:98, 1957.

1362. Fritz, M.H.: The Scarred Corneas of Alaska, *Alaska Med* 1: 116–117, 1959.

1363. Thygeson, P., and Dawson, C.R.: Ophthalmological Problems of the American Indian, *Trans Pacif Coast Otoophthal Soc,* 1959, pp 39–62.

1364. Schwartz, J.R., et al: Status of Tonometry Surveys as a Source of Epidemiologic Data, *Public Health Rep* 82:582 (July) 1967.

1365. Portney, G.L.: The Treatment of Endemic Pterygium in the Navajo, abstracted, *Proc 3rd Joint Meet of the Clin Soc and Commissioned Officers Ass USPHS,* San Francisco, Calif (March) 1968, p 28.

1366. Chen, J.; Rosenbaum, L.J.; and Hoshiwara, I.: Unusual Manifestations of Uveitis in Southwestern American Indians, abstracted, *Proc 4th Joint Meet of the Clin Soc and Commissioned Officers Ass USPHS,* Boston (June) 1969, p 15.

1367. Hoshiwara, I.; Chen, J.; and Rosenbaum, L.J.: The Use of Automatic Data and Processing in the Outpatient Eye Clinic at the Phoenix Indian Hospital, abstracted, *Proc 4th Joint Meet of the Clin Soc and Commissioned Officers Ass USPHS,* Boston (June) 1969, p 70.

1368. Levy, W.J., et al: A Study of the Refractive State of a Group of American Pueblo Indians, *Rocky Mountain Med J* 66:40–42 (Sept) 1969.

1369. Portney, G.L.: Bare Sclera, Scleral Cautery, and Corticosteroid Therapy of Endemic Pterygium in the Navajo Indians, *Amer J Ophthal* 67:759–761 (May) 1969.

1370. Rosenbaum, L.J.; Chen, J.; and Hoshiwara, I.: Non-Traumatic Leukomas in Southwestern Indians, abstracted, *Proc 4th Joint Meet of the Clin Soc and Commissioned Officers Ass USPHS,* Boston (June) 1969, p 15.

B. EAR

1371. Moodie, R.L.: Deafness Among Ancient Californian Indians, *Bull Southern Calif Acad Sci* 28 (pt 3):46–49, 1929.

1372. Many Children Attend Alaska EENT Clinics, *Alaska's Health* 11:6 (Aug) 1954.

1373. Fritz, M.H.: Natural History of Ear Disease in Arctic Villages, Alaska, abstracted, *Sci in Alaska*, Proc 7th Alaskan Sci Conf (1956), AAAS, Alaska Div, pp 96–97.

1374. Ear, Nose, and Throat Special Demonstration Project Initiated, *Alaska's Health* 14:1–2 (Aug) 1957.

1375. Otitis Media Prophylaxis Used for Indian Children, *Public Health Rep* 74:247 (March) 1959.

1376. Ensign, P.R.; Urbanich, E.M.; and Morgan, M.: Prophylaxis of Otitis Media in an Indian Population, *Amer J Public Health* 50:195–196 (Feb) 1960.

1377. Dolowitz, D.A., et al: Hearing Rehabilitation with Modified Radical Mastoidectomy, *Texas J Med* 9:962–967 (Oct) 1963.

1378. Brody, J.A.: Notes on the Epidemiology of Draining Ears and Hearing Loss in Alaska with Comment on Future Studies and Control Measures, *Alaska Med* 6:1–4, 1964.

1379. Cambon, K.; Galbraith, J.D.; and Kong, G.: Middle-Ear Disease in Indians of the Mount Currie Reservation, British Columbia, *Canad Med Ass J* 93:1301 (Dec) 1965.

1380. Johnson, R.L.: Chronic Otitis Media in Schoolage Navajo Indians, abstracted, *Proc 1st Joint Meet of the Clin Soc and Commissioned Officers Ass USPHS*, Baltimore, Md (May) 1966, p 7.

1381. Justice, J.: Audiometric Screening by Indian Volunteers, abstracted, *Proc 1st Joint Meet of the Clin Soc and Commissioned Officers Ass USPHS*, Baltimore, Md (May) 1966, p. 55.

1382. Johnson, R.L.: Chronic Otitis Media in School Age Navajo Indians, *Laryngoscope* 77:1990–1995 (May) 1967.

1383. Petrakis, N.L.; Molonhon, K.T.; and Tepper, D.J.: Cerumen in American Indians: Genetic Implication of Sticky and Dry Types, *Science* 158:1192–1193 (Dec) 1967.

1384. Zonis, R.D.: Chronic Otitis Media in the Southwestern American Indian, I: Prevalence, *Arch Otolaryng* 88:360–365 (Oct) 1968; and II: Immunologic Factors, *Arch Otolaryng* 88:366–369 (Oct) 1968.

1385. Jaffe, B.: The Incidence of Ear Diseases in the Navajo Indians, *Laryngoscope* 79:2126–2134 (Dec) 1969.

1386. Petrakis, N.L.: Dry Cerumen—A Prevalent Genetic Trait Among American Indians, *Nature* 22:1080–1081 (June 14) 1969.

1387. Zonis, R.D.: Meckel's Cartilage Remnant? *Laryngoscope* 79: 2012–2015 (Nov) 1969.

XXI. DENTAL STUDIES AND PROBLEMS

1388. Allen, W.A.: Indians Immune to Pyorrhea, *Item Interest* 22: 251, 1900.

1389. Price, W.A.: New Light on the Etiology of Facial Deformity and Dental Irregularities from Field Studies Among Eskimos and Indians in Various Stages of Modernization, *J Dent Res* 14:229–230, 1934.

1390. Price, W.A.: Relation of Nutrition to Dental Caries Among Eskimos and Indians in Alaska and Northern Canada, *J Dent Res* 14:227–229, 1934.

1391. Steggerda, M., and Hill, T.J.: Incidence of Dental Caries Among Maya and Navajo Indians, *J Dent Res* 15:233–242, 1936.

1392. Arnim, S.S.; Aberle, S.B.D.; and Pitney, E.H.: Dental Changes in Group of Pueblo Indian Children, *J Amer Dent Ass* 24: 478–480, 1937.

1393. Klein, E.: Dental Caries, *Public Health Bull*, No. 239 (Dec) 1937.

1394. Nelson, C.T.: The Teeth of the Indians of Pecos Pueblo, *Amer J Phys Anthrop* 23:261–293, 1938.

1395. Report of Committee on Indian Affairs of the Canadian Dental Association, *J Canad Dent Ass* 5:34, 1939.

1396. Colquitt, W.T., and Webb, C.H.: Dental Diseases in Aboriginal Group, *Tri-State Med J* 12:2414–2417, 1940.

1397. Foster, L.W.: Dental Conditions in White and Indian Children in Northern Wisconsin, *J Amer Dent Ass* 29:2251–2255, 1942.

1398. Livermore, A.R.: Vitamins and Minerals in the Prevention of Caries: Report of 2-year Experiment with 84 Children, *Dent Survey* 18:1169, 1942.

1399. Steggerda, M., and Hill, T.J.: Eruption Time of Teeth Among Whites, Negroes, and Indians, *Amer J Orthodont* 28:361–370, 1942.

1400. Webb, G.H.: Dental Abnormalities, *Amer J Orthodont* 30:474–486, 1944.

1401. Heller, C.A.: Food and Dental Health, *Alaska's Health* 4:4–5 (Dec) 1946.

1402. *Oral Health Program of the Division of Indian Health: Annual Report*, US Public Health Serv, Div of Indian Health, 1957.

1403. Dahlberg, A.A., and Menegaz-Bock, R.M.: Emergence of the Permanent Teeth in Pima Indian Children, *J Dent Res* 37:1123–1140 (Nov–Dec) 1958.

1404. *Oral Health Program of the Division of Indian Health: Annual Report*, US Public Health Serv, Div of Indian Health, 1958.

1405. *Dental Services for Indians, Annual Report*, US Public Health Serv, Div of Indian Health, 1959.

1406. *Dental Services for Indians: Annual Report*, US Public Health Serv, Div of Indian Health, 1960.

1407. Greene, J.C.: Oral Hygiene and Periodontal Disease, *J Oklahoma Med Ass* 53:503–509 (July) 1960.

1408. Parfitt, G.J.: A Survey of the Oral Health of Navajo Indian Children, *Arch Oral Biol* 1:193–205 (Jan) 1960.

1409. *Dental Services for Indians: Annual Report*, US Public Health Serv, Div of Indian Health, 1961.

1410. Spruce, G.B., Jr.: American Indians as Dental Patients, *Public Health Rep* 76:1059–1062 (Dec) 1961.

1411. *Dental Services for Indians: Annual Report*, US Public Health Serv, Div of Indian Health, 1962.

1412. *Dental Services for Indians: Annual Report*, US Public Health Serv, Div of Indian Health, 1963.

1413. *Report of Presentations to the Council on Federal Dental Services of the American Dental Association*, US Public Health Serv (Jan 7–9) 1963.

1414. *Dental Services for Indians: Annual Report*, US Public Health Serv, Div of Indian Health, 1964.

1415. *Dentistry for Indians and Alaska Natives, A Report to the American Dental Association*, US Public Health Serv, Div of Indian Health (Aug) 1964.

1416. *Dentistry in Alaska, Award-Winning Dental Team*, TIC (Sept) 1964.

1417. Merrill, R.G.: Occlusal Anomalous Tubercles on Premolars of Alaskan Eskimos and Indians, *Oral Surg* 17:484–496 (April) 1964.

1418. Myers, S.E.: Dental Hygiene for American Indians, *J Amer Dent Hygienists Ass*, vol 38 (No. 4) 1964.

1419. Archard, H.O.; Heck, J.W.; and Stanley, H.R.: Focal Epithelial Hyperplasia: An Unusual Oral Mucosal Lesion Found in Indian Children, *Oral Surg* 20:201–212 (Aug) 1965.

1420. *Dental Services for American Indians and Alaska Natives: Annual Report*, US Public Health Serv, Div of Indian Health, 1965.

1421. *Oral Health Program of the Division of Indian Health: Annual Report*, US Public Health Serv, Div of Indian Health, 1965–1966.

1422. Abramowitz, J.: Expanded Functions for Dental Assistants: A Preliminary Study, *J Amer Dent Ass* 72:386–391 (Feb) 1966.

1423. Birch, R.C.: The Efficient Utilization of Auxiliary Dental Personnel—A Division of Indian Health Team Approach, abstracted, *Proc 1st Joint Meet of the Clin Soc and Commissioned Officers Ass USPHS*, Baltimore, Md (May) 1966, p 54.

1424. Curzon, M.E.: Dentistry Among Canadian Indians, *Dental Mag Oral Topics* 83:132–133, 1966.

1425. *Dental Services for American Indians and Alaska Natives: Annual Report*, US Public Health Serv, Div of Indian Health, Publ 1550, 1966.

1426. Flynn, L.R., and Heck, J.W.: Natal and Neonatal Teeth: A Study Among the Indians of Southwestern US, abstracted, *Proc 1st Joint Meet of the Clin Soc and Commissioned Officers Ass USPHS*, Baltimore, Md (May) 1966, p 6.

1427. Hicks, M.A.: A Study of the Eruption Pattern of the Permanent Dentition in Navajo Children, abstracted, *Proc 1st Joint Meet of the Clin Soc and Commissioned Officers Ass USPHS*, Baltimore, Md (May) 1966, p 6.

1428. Mayhall, J.T.: A Study of Natal and Neonatal Teeth Among the Tlinget Indians, abstracted, *Proc 1st Joint Meet of the Clin Soc and Commissioned Officers Ass USPHS*, Baltimore, Md (May) 1966, p 6.

1429. Morris, D.H.: Morphological Analysis and Age in the Permanent Dentition of Young American Indians, *Amer J Phys Anthrop* 75:91–96 (July) 1966.

1430. Nasi, J.H.: Acute Gingival Disease in the Young, abstracted, *Proc 1st Joint Meet of the Clin Soc and Commissioned Officers Ass USPHS*, Baltimore, Md (May) 1966, p 6.

1431. *Report on the Conference of the Division of Indian Health Dental Services Branch with the Council on Federal Dental Services of the American Dental Association*, US Public Health Serv, Div of Indian Health (March) 1966.

1432. Ship, I.I.: Dental Caries Incidence in North and South Dakota Indian School Children During 30 Years, *J Dent Res* 45:359–363 (March–April) 1966.

1433. Ship, I.I.: *Nutrition and Dental Caries: Effects of Phosphate Supplements*, Amer Ass Adv Sci, Publ 81, 1966, pp 109–151.

1434. Birch, R.C.: The Role of the Dental Assistant in the Dental Program for Indians, *Dent Assist* 36:14–19 (May–June) 1967.

1435. Birch, R.C.: The Role of the Dental Assistant in the Dental Program for Indians, abstracted, *Proc 2nd Joint Meet of the Clin Soc and Commissioned Officers Ass USPHS*, Atlanta, Ga (May) 1967, p 3.

1436. *The Dental Health Program for American Indians, Eskimos, and Aleuts*, US Public Health Serv, Div of Indian Health, Publ 1585, 1967.

1437. *Dental Services for American Indians and Alaska Natives: Annual Report*, US Public Health Serv, Div of Indian Health, Publ 1724, 1967.

1438. Fallows, R.: The Extent of Contamination in the Dental Operatory by the Water and Air Spray, abstracted, *Proc 2nd Joint Meet of the Clin Soc and Commissioned Officers Ass USPHS*, Atlanta, Ga (May) 1967, p 47.

1439. Mayhall, J.T.: Natal and Neonatal Teeth Among the Tlingit Indians, *J Dent Res* 46:748–749 (July–Aug) 1967.

1440. Morris, D.H.: Maxillary Premolar Variation Among the Papago Indians, *J Dent Res* 46:736–738 (July–Aug) 1967.

1441. *Preventive Orthodontics and Limited Treatment Procedures—Manual*, US Public Health Serv, Publ 1653, 1967.

1442. *Report on the Conference with the Council on Federal Dental Services of the American Dental Association*, US Public Health Serv, Div of Indian Health (Aug) 1967.

1443. Cumming, J.R.: Bush Dentistry, 1968 Style, *Alaska Med* 10: 71–75, 1968.

1444. Curry, L.: Complications of Supernumerary Fourth Molars: A Review of the Literature and Report of a Case, abstracted, *Proc 3rd Joint Meet of the Clin Soc and Commissioned Officers Ass USPHS*, San Francisco, Calif (March) 1968, p 15.

1445. *Dental Assistant Training Standard Course Outline*, US Public Health Serv, Div of Indian Health (May) 1968.

1446. *Dental Services for American Indians and Alaska Natives: Annual Report*, US Public Health Serv, Div of Indian Health, Publ 1870, 1968.

1447. Grewe, J.M., et al: Prevalence of Malocclusion in Chippewa Indian Children, *J Dent Res* 47:302–305, 1968.

1448. McClellan, T.E., and Cox, J.E.: Description and Evaluation of Dentist–Dental Assistant Teaching Team Training in Efficient Dental Practice Management, *J Amer Dent Ass* 76:549–553 (March) 1968.

1449. *Report of the Conference of the Division of Indian Health Dental Services Branch with the Federal Dental Services of the American Dental Association*, US Public Health Serv, Div of Indian Health, 1968.

1450. Boggs, D.C.: Simple Technique for Treating Non-Vital Deciduous Teeth—A Study, *North-West Dentistry* 48 (March–April) 1969.

1451. Butts, J.E.: The Alaska Area Native Health Service Dental Program, *Alaska Med* 11:24–25, 1969.

1452. *Dental Services for American Indians and Alaska Natives: Annual Report*, US Public Health Serv, Health Serv and Mental Health Administration, Indian Health Serv, 1969.

1453. Fasano, R.J., et al: Incidence of Dental Disease Among the Navajo Indians of Monument Valley, Utah, *J Dent Res* 48: 328 (March–April) 1969.

1454. Malarkey, H.F.: Malocclusion in the Primary Dentition Among the Navajo, abstracted, *Proc 4th Joint Meet of the Clin Soc and Commissioned Officers Ass USPHS*, Boston (June) 1969, p 61.

1455. *Preventive Periodontics: Manual for Dental Prophylaxis and Related Health Education*, US Public Health Serv (July) 1969.

1456. *Report on the Conference of the Division of Indian Health Dental Services Branch with the Council on Federal Dental Services of the American Dental Association*, US Public Health Serv, Health Serv and Mental Health Administration, Indian Health Serv (Jan) 1969.

1457. Turner, C.G., and Cadien, J.D.: Dental Chipping in Aleuts, Eskimos, and Indians, *Amer J Phys Anthrop* 31:303–310 (Nov) 1969.

1458. *Dental Intern Training Program and Manual: Gallup Indian Medical Center*, US Public Health Serv, Health Serv and Mental Health Administration, Indian Health Serv (July) 1969–(June) 1970.

1459. *Dental Intern Training Program and Manual: PHS Alaska Native Medical Center*, US Public Health Serv, Health Serv and Mental Health Administration, Indian Health Serv (July) 1969–(June) 1970.

1460. *Dental Intern Training Program and Manual: PHS Indian Hospital Fort Defiance, Arizona*, US Public Health Serv, Health Serv and Mental Health Administration, Indian Health Serv (July) 1969–(June) 1970.

XXII. MISCELLANEOUS TOPICS

A. MALNUTRITION AND VITAMIN DEFICIENCIES

1461. Pijoan, M.; Elkin, C.A.; and Eslinger, C.O.: Ascorbic Acid Deficiency Among Papago Indians, *J Nutr* 25:491–496, 1942.

1462. Corrigan, R.S.C.: Scurvy in a Cree Indian, *Canad Med Ass J* 54:380–383 (April) 1946.

1463. Levine, V.E.: The Epidemic of Scurvy Among the Indians of the Omaha Tribe, 1844–1845, *Amer J Dig Dis* 22:294–295 (Oct) 1955.

1464. Schaefer, O.: Medical Observations and Problems in the Canadian Arctic, II: Nutrition and Nutritional Deficiencies, *Canad Med Ass J* 81:386–393 (Sept) 1959.

1465. Wilcox, E.B., and Grimes, M.: Gingivitis—Ascorbic Acid Deficiency in the Navajo, I: Ascorbic Acid in White-cell–Platelet Fraction of Blood, *J Nutr* 74:352–356 (Aug) 1961.

1466. Wolfe, C.B.: Kwashiorkor on the Navajo Indian Reservation, *Henry Ford Hosp Med Bull* 9:566–569, 1961.

1467. McDonald, B.S.: Gingivitis—Ascorbic Acid Deficiency in the Navajo, III: Dietary Aspects, *J Amer Diet Ass* 43:332–335 (Oct) 1963.

1468. Demers, P., et al: An Epidemiological Study of Infantile Scurvy in Canada, 1961–1963, *Canad Med Ass J* 93:573–576 (Sept) 1965.

1469. Chabon, R.S.: Kwashiorkor in a Navajo Indian Child, abstracted, *Proc 2nd Joint Meet of the Clin Soc and Commissioned Officers Ass USPHS*, Atlanta, Ga (May) 1967, p 1.

1470. Van Duzen, J., et al: Protein and Calorie Malnutrition Among Pre-School Navajo Indian Children, *Amer J Clin Nutr* 22:1362–1370 (Oct) 1969.

B. TRAUMA AND ACCIDENTS

1471. Courville, C.B.: Cranial Injuries Among Indians of North America: Preliminary Report, *Bull Los Angeles Neurol Soc* 13:181–219, 1948.

1472. Haldeman, J.C.: "Violent and Accidental Deaths as a Health Problem in Alaska," in *Sci in Alaska*, Proc 2nd Alaskan Sci Conf (1951), AAAS, Alaska Div, pp 103–107.

1473. Schmitt, N., and Barclay, W.S.: Accidental Deaths Among West Coast Indians, *Canad J Public Health* 53:409–412 (Oct) 1962.

1474. Schmitt, N.; Hole, L.W.; and Barclay, W.S.: Accidental

Deaths Among British Columbia Indians, *Canad Med Ass J* 94:228–234 (Jan) 1966.

1475. Brown, R.C.: Epidemiology of Accidents Among the Navajo Indian, abstracted, *Proc 3rd Joint Meet of the Clin Soc and Commissioned Officers Ass USPHS*, San Francisco, Calif (March) 1968, p 37.

1476. Boyd, D.L.; Maynard, J.E.; and Hammes, L.M.: Accident Mortality in Alaska, 1958–1962, *Arch Environ Health* 17:101–106 (July) 1968.

C. OTHER MISCELLANEOUS PUBLICATIONS

1477. Daniel, Z.T.: Amputation of the Leg of a Full-Blooded Sioux Indian, *Intl J Surg* 4:54, 1891.

1478. Stirling, M.W.: *Snake Bites and Hopi Snake Dance*, Smithsonian Inst, Publ 3651, 1942, pp 551–555.

1479. Kovacs, L., et al: Acute Disseminated Lupus Erythematosus in a North American Indian Girl, *Canad Med Ass J* 74:552–556 (April) 1956.

1480. Richey, D.F.: Observations of an Obese Population, abstracted, *Proc 1st Joint Meet of the Clin Soc and Commissioned Officers Ass USPHS*, Baltimore, Md (May) 1966, p 21.

1481. Sparger, C.F.: Straight Pin Ingestion in an American Indian Boarding School, *Maryland Med J* 17:43–47 (Nov) 1968.

1482. Johnson, D.G.: Conference on Increasing Representation in Medical Schools of Afro-Americans, Mexican-Americans, and American Indians, *J Med Educ* 44:710–711 (Aug) 1969.

1483. Sparger, C.F.: Problems in the Management of Rattlesnake Bites, *Arch Surg* 98:13–18 (Jan) 1969.

AUTHOR INDEX

Aach, D., 710
Abbott, K.H., 1000
Abbott, W.A., 814
Aberle, S.B.D., 57, 92, 1137, 1138, 1142, 1204, 1392
Abraham, S., 1271
Abramowitz, J., 1422
Adair, J., 300, 519, 535
Adami, G.C., 171
Adams, G.S., 1348, 1349
Adams, M.S., 1156, 1157, 1188, 1191, 1196, 1197
Adams, T., 139
Adams, W.R., 68
Adamson, J.D., 692, 693
Addison, P., 797
Albrecht, C.E., 484, 494, 661
Aldous, H.E., 1190
Allen, C., 681
Allen, G., 953
Allen, W.A., 1388
Alley, R., 841
Alley, R.D., 780
Allison, A.C., 1164

Alter, A.J., 515
Andersen, K.L., 140, 141
Anderson, C.M., 1096
Anderson, F.N., 1026
Anderson, M.W., 613
Andrews, E., 227
Andros, F., 18, 231
Anthony, B.F., 774, 775, 779
Archard, H.O., 1419
Armstrong, F.B., 911
Arnim, S.S., 1392
Aronson, C.F., 868, 871, 890
Aronson, J.D., 58, 63, 829, 842, 850, 852, 855, 856, 868, 871, 876, 883, 890, 971
Arthur, G., 1115
Ashburn, F.D., 286
Ashburn, P.M., 54

Babbott, F.L., Jr., 566, 674, 675, 677, 678
Babbott, J.G., 674, 675
Babero, B.B., 993
Bahl, I.E., 542

Bailey, F.L., 479, 1148
Baizerman, M., 603
Baker, J.L., 1052
Bales, R.F., 1053
Ballestero, R.J., 1193
Balsamo, P., 1168
Bang, G., 1337, 1339
Barclay, W.S., 1473, 1474
Barker, W.T., 1131
Barnett, H.E., 287
Barton, S., 1020
Barzelatto, J., 1344
Bass, W.M., 199
Beamish, W.E., 891
Beaugrand-Champagne, A., 61
Bebchuck, W., 1303
Beck, C.W., 207
Becker, D.A., 690, 941
Beer, A.E., 1155
Belloc, N.B., 1361
Belshaw, C.S., 1050
Benedict, A.L., 240, 439
Benedict, R., 1161
Bennett, K.A., 209
Bennett, P.H., 768, 1172, 1249–1251,
     1254, 1279, 1298–1300, 1325, 1327
Bentzen, R.C., 162
Berg, L.E., 1158
Berger, L.S., 1230
Best, E.W.R., 310
Birch, R.C., 1423, 1434, 1435
Birt, A.R., 1229
Bissell, G.P., 1127
Biswell, R., 758
Bivens, M.D., 1013
Bjork, J., 1034
Blackwell, R.O., 1292
Blake, J.D., 658
Bleyer, A., 1179
Blomquist, E.T., 872
Blumberg, B.S., 1164
Bock, G.E., 604
Bödecker, C.F., 165
Boedeker, M.T., 127
Boggs, D.C., 1019, 1450
Bone, M., 772
Bonehill, B., 1290
Borden, W.C., 86
Bosley, B., 113
Boteler, W.C., 133
Bourke, J.G., 1045
Bow, M.R., 693
Bowman, C.R., 629

Boyd, D.L., 1476
Boyer, L.B., 1118, 1120
Boynton, R.E., 450
Braasch, W.F., 351
Brailsford, A.M., 260
Branton, B.J., 351
Braude, F.F., 772
Brenneman, G., 786, 787, 1224
Brewer, I.W., 799
Britton, W.B., 525
Brody, J.A., 785, 1378
Bromberg, W., 1091
Brooke, M.M., 689
Brooks, H., 258, 265
Brothwell, D.R., 210
Brown, C.V., 1290
Brown, G.W., 1258, 1290
Brown, J.E., 1297
Brown, M., 992
Brown, R.C., 1475
Brown, W.C., 806
Bryans, B., 1152
Buchan, D.J., 926
Bull, H.R., 795
Bunim, J.J., 1171, 1233, 1236, 1240,
     1241
Burch, T.A., 1171, 1172, 1233, 1235,
     1236, 1240–1242, 1245, 1249–1251,
     1254, 1279, 1298–1300, 1325, 1327
Burns, H.A., 814, 815, 821
Bushnell, G.E., 789
Butler, J.J., 458
Butts, J.E., 1451
Byers, W.G.M., 738

Cadien, J.D., 1457
Cady, L.D., 749
Cambon, K., 1379
Cameron, C.M., Jr., 358
Cameron, T.W.M., 687, 688, 990
Canavan, M.M., 181
Cark, W., 928
Carlile, W.K., 592, 975
Carney, R.E., 1119
Caron, M., 880
Carpenter, C.W., 1152
Carpenter, E.S., 1054
Carpenter, T.M., 102
Carrington, T.S., 88
Carroll, N.V., 1334
Carswell, J.A., 838
Casey, J.C., 543
Casselman, E., 605

Chabon, R.S., 1309, 1469
Chance, N.A., 157
Chapman, F.H., 200
Chen, J., 1366, 1367, 1370
Chesky, J., 292
Chesley, A.J., 351, 449, 731
Chin, T.D.Y., 697
Christensen, C., 1297
Church, G.M., 1212
Clairmont, D.H., 1055
Clark, W., 573
Clement, E., 1122
Clifford, N.J., 1275
Clifford, S., 203
Cobb, C.M., 43
Cobb, J.C., 750
Cocking, R.R., 1042
Coddington, F.L., 983
Coffey, M.F., 137
Coffin, R., 115
Cogswell, W.F., 374
Cohen, B.M., 1264, 1314
Cohen, F.S., 348
Cohen, J.J., 1259, 1260
Collier, J., 266, 455
Collins, R.J., 809
Collins, R.N., 955
Colquitt, W.T., 1396
Colyar, A.B., 552, 553, 567
Comess, L.J., 1201, 1298–1300, 1331
Comstock, G.W., 895, 899, 905, 907,
  922, 924, 973
Congdon, R.T., 173
Connel, M.F., 658
Conroy, E., 771
Cook, S.F., 51, 276
Corrigan, C., 1181
Corrigan, R.S.C., 62, 1462
Coulter, P.O., 630
Courville, C.B., 193, 1000, 1471
Covarrubias, E., 1344
Covino, B.G., 139
Cowen, R.D., 1004
Cox, J.E., 1448
Crain, K.C., 469
Cressman, L.S., 190
Crile, G.W., 136
Crockett, B.N., 72
Crouch, J.H., 735, 816
Cullinson, S., 676
Cumming, G.R., 150
Cumming, J.R., 1443
Cummings, M.M., 897

Cummins, S.L., 810
Curley, R.T., 1064
Currier, 1130
Curry, L., 1444
Curzon, J.A., 1194
Curzon, M.E., 1194, 1424

Dafoe, C.S., 908
Dahlberg, A.A., 95, 1403
Dahlstrom, A.W., 849, 862, 865
Daniel, Z.T., 1477
Danielson, B.D., 1301
Darby, G.E., 267
Darby, W.J., 111
Darling, D., 222
Davis, B.M., 499
Davis, H., 817
Davis, R., 873
Davis, T.R.A., 708, 709, 987
Dawson, C.R., 750, 754, 1363
Day, E.K., 489, 495
Deacon, W.E., 614
Dean, J.D., 512
Decker, A., 1259
DeForest, J.W., 19
DeLien, H., 496, 862, 864, 865, 932
Dellinger, S.C., 101
Demers, P., 1468
DeMontigny, L.H., 631
Denninger, H.S., 169, 170, 178, 183
Detal, C.S., 299
Deuschle, K.W., 300, 519, 535, 569,
  892, 896, 918
Devereux, G., 1027, 1048, 1077, 1086,
  1089, 1094, 1112–1114, 1145, 1146,
  1149, 1206
Dickie, W.M., 269
Diddams, A., 920
Dietz, J., 729
Dillenberg, H., 778
Dixon, G.L., 1263
Dobson, P.M., 705
Dodson, M.W., 782
Doeblin, T.D., 1331A, 1332
Dolowitz, D.A., 1190, 1377
Dowler, B., 436
Downey, J.L., 1303
Dozier, E.P., 1062
Drevets, C.C., 1317, 1319
Driver, H.E., 2
Dubois, J., 869
Duffy, J., 726
Dufner, F.J., 930

Duggan, J.W., 1357
Duncan, A.C., 105
Dunham, C.L., 1231
Dunham, E.C., 135
Durham, D.G., 1353
Durham, W.F., 152
Dustin, U.L., 854
Duxrury, J., 36

Eagan, C.J., 148
Eastman, C.A., 248, 444
Eaton, R.D.P., 934, 935, 937
Ede, M.C., 1322
Eder, H.A., 1270
Edwards, A.M., 911, 1338
Edwards, L.B., 922
Eilers, P.G., 742
Elett, R., 1287
Elkin, C.A., 765, 1205, 1461
Elmendorf, W.W., 1095
Elsea, W.R., 783
Elsner, R.W., 141, 142
Emerling, F.G., 1332
Emerson, H., 254
Emmons, G.T., 342
Englebert, E., 218
Ensign, P.R., 1376
Eslinger, C.O., 1461
Evans, J.P., 20
Everett, M.A., 1227
Evonuk, E., 145, 147, 148

Fahy, A., 319
Falconer, W.L., 67
Fallows, R., 1438
Farber, E.M., 1228
Fasano, R.J., 1453
Fehlinger, H., 244
Feldman, F.F., 821
Fellows, F.S., 825
Felsman, F.W., 930
Ferguson, F.D., 38
Ferguson, F.N., 1067
Ferguson, R.G., 811, 812, 823, 826, 858
Fieldsteel, A.H., 697
Finch, C.A., 1173
Findley, D., 578
Fischer, S., 1092
Fisher, A.K., 171
Fleming, H.C., 252, 253
Flemming, A.S., 526
Fleshman, J.K., 332, 1260

Flood, F., 923
Flower, W.H., 83
Flynn, L.R., 1195, 1426
Foard, F.T., 291, 486, 487, 870
Forster, W.G., 747
Fortuine, R., 4, 786–788
Foster, A., 1123
Foster, E., 524
Foster, L.W., 1397
Foster, S.O., 728, 752, 753
Fournelle, F., 676
Fournelle, H.J., 681
Fowler, D.M., 1361
Fox, C., 798
Fox, H., 1226
Fox, L.W., 730, 736
Frank, I., 671
Frank, M.L., 765
Frankenhauser, E., 74
Fraser, C.A.M., 776
Fraser, R.I., 913–915
Frederiksen, M.J., 1291
Freestone, A., 615
Freimark, L.G., 1307
French, F.S., 512
French, J.G., 1217
Fritz, M.H., 1351–1353, 1355, 1359, 1362, 1373
Frohman, L.A., 1332
Fry, G.F., 218
Fulmer, H.S., 1276

Gaddes, W.H., 1036
Gaenslen, E.C., 916
Galbraith, J.D., 1379
Gallina, J.N., 593
Garcia, C., 1155
Gard, S., 707
Garth, T.R., 1177
Gaumand, E., 866
Geare, R.I., 250
Geary, J.M., 964
Geller, A., 1261
Gentles, E.W., 893
Genuth, S.M., 1324
Gerken, E.A., 466, 467
Gerloff, R.K., 695
Gerrard, J.W., 668
Gibson, H.V., 696
Giebink, G.S., 779
Giglioli, G., 979
Gilbert, J., 1265, 1267, 1272
Gilbert, M.E., 832

Gilbert, R., 632
Gill, G.D., 964
Gilliam, A.G., 1006
Gillick, D.W., 818
Gilmore, M.R., 1139
Githens, J.H., 1288
Gitlitz, I., 672
Glisan, R., 224
Goble, M.G., 1193
Godfrey, G.C.M., 1134
Gofton, J.P., 1234, 1238, 1239, 1243, 1246, 1247, 1252
Goldstein, M.S., 195, 196, 216
Goodwin, M.H., 679
Gordan, B.L., 66
Gordon, J.E., 674, 675, 677, 678
Cortler, S.M., 1164
Gottmann, A.W., 305
Graham, J.B., 794
Graham-Cumming, G., 79, 1218–1220
Grant, R.B., 1167
Grauer, F., 1228
Graves, T.D., 1065
Gray, C.G., 1232, 1338
Greenberg, L., 658
Greene, J.C., 1407
Gregg, J.B., 202, 203
Grenfell, W.T., 45
Grewe, J.M., 1447
Griffin, B.I., 154
Griffin, W., 554
Grimes, M., 1465
Grinnell, F., 39, 229
Grinnell, G.B., 1135
Grumbles, L.C., 965
Gurunanjappa, B.S., 100, 1221
Guthrie, M.C., 255, 259, 732

Haas, L.E., 513
Hadley, J.N., 297, 496, 932
Haldeman, J.C., 490, 1472
Hallowell, A.I., 1025
Halton, W.L., 184
Hamer, J.H., 1061
Hamlin, H., 345
Hammel, H.T., 146
Hammer, H.R., 1080, 1081
Hammes, L.M., 1277, 1476
Hampton, J.E., 1286
Hancock, J.C., 268, 743
Hanna, B.L., 95
Hanna, L., 751

Hannon, J.P., 145, 147
Hanson, M.L., 924
Hanson, W.C., 153–155
Hardenberg, W., 480
Hardy, A.V., 670
Hardy, E.R., 1168
Hardy, J.D., 1350
Harris, R.L., 1198
Hart, J.S., 144
Hatfield, R.E., 1357
Havighurst, R.J., 1116
Hawthorne, H.B., 1050
Hayes, M., 470
Hayman, C.R., 138, 663, 884, 1207, 1208
Hayworth, D.D., 1068
Heagerty, J.J., 721
Healy, G.R., 940, 942
Heath, D.B., 1059
Heck, J.W., 1419, 1426
Hefferman, W.T., 33
Heller, C.A., 122, 125, 128, 129, 1401
Henderson, N.E., 1035
Henk, M.L., 1074
Henry, R.E., 1325, 1333
Herbert, F.A., 762, 952
Herdman, R.C., 777
Hermansen, L., 141
Herxheimer, H., 1257
Hesse, F.G., 114, 315, 1294
Hetherington, H.W., 834
Hickey, J.L.S., 580
Hicks, M.A., 1427
Hilbert, H., 450
Hildes, J.A., 302, 527, 536, 706, 948, 950
Hill, R.H., 1255
Hill, T.J., 1391, 1399
Hill, W.W., 1178
Hirsch, A., 158
Hirsch, J.S., 110
Hislop, D.M.C., 1305
Hodge, F.W., 246
Hoffman, F.L., 261, 452, 996
Holder, A.B., 236, 1128, 1132
Hole, L.W., 1474
Holmes, R.H., 1160
Holzhueter, A.M., 202, 203
Honess, R.E., 684
Honigmann, I., 1047
Honigmann, J.J., 657, 1047
Hopla, C.E., 966, 967

Horton, D., 1046
Hoshiwara, I., 755, 756, 759, 1366, 1367, 1370
Hoskins, D.D., 1162, 1163
Hoyt, E.E., 1031
Hrdlička, A., 60, 94, 177, 186, 243, 245, 249, 251, 263, 802, 1140
Hudgins, H.A., 545
Hunter, J.D., 11, 12
Huntley, B.E., 970
Hursch, L.M., 112
Hutchinson, W., 801

Innis, H.A., 349
Irving, L., 142, 143, 151

Jackson, H.C., 528
Jaffe, B., 1018, 1199, 1385
Jamieson, S.M., 1050
Jarcho, S., 204, 208
Jenness, D., 311
Johnson, C.C., 601
Johnson, D.G., 1043, 1482
Johnson, J.E., 1318
Johnson, M.W., 1016
Johnson, R.L., 1380, 1382
Johnson, W., 1104, 1105
Jones, C.F., 96
Jones, H., 46
Jones, J., 27
Jones, J.A., 1169
Jones, L.R., 843
Jones, M., 296
Jonz, W.W., 596
Jordan, S.W., 1021
Joseph, A., 292, 1088
Joslin, E.P., 1312, 1313, 1315
Josselyn, J., 7
Julianelle, L.A., 746
Justice, J., 1381
Justice, J.W., 665, 1015

Kanner, L., 1348, 1349
Kartchner, M.M., 77, 78
Kartman, L., 954, 956
Keast, T.J., 1101
Keefer, F.J., 1341
Kelln, E.E., 211
Kelly, J.J., Jr., 1270
Kemmerer, A.R., 110
Kern, M., 1124
Kester, E.R., 138
Kester, F.E., 312, 663, 1208, 1277

King, J.C., 1136
Klebs, A.C., 803
Klein, E., 1393
Kleinman, H., 769, 772
Klopper, B., 1118
Kluckhohn, C., 98
Kneeland, T., 225, 437
Knight, J.L., 597, 620
Kong, G., 1379
Koritzer, R.T., 213
Korns, J.H., 833
Kositchek, R.J., 1274
Kovacs, L., 1479
Kraus, B.S., 296, 1182, 1185
Kravetz, R.E., 316, 1296
Krogman, W.M., 91
Kronenberg, B., 1360
Krulish, E., 42, 247, 441
Krush, T.P., 1034, 1100
Krutz, G., 755, 756, 759
Kuhm, H.W., 171
Kunce, J., 1122
Kunitz, S.J., 1311
Kuttner, R.E., 1066, 1306

LaBarre, W., 1093
Lackman, D.B., 702, 704
LaHontan, 8
Lake, A.D., 241
Lam, R.C., 1293
Landes, R., 1085
Lane, R.F., 894
Langford, H.G., 1151
Lantis, M., 555, 1029
Larsell, O., 64, 190
Larson, J.A., 70
Lasersohn, W., 680
Lawler, D., 760
Lawrence, J.S., 1248
Lawson, R.N., 1004
Lear, L., 889
Lee, B.J., 997, 998
Lee, J.F., 637
Leer, R.H., 1356
Lees, B., 581
Leggett, E.A., 874
Leigh, R.W., 163
Leighton, A.H., 284, 1037, 1038, 1087, 1090
Leighton, D.C., 1087, 1090
Lemert, E.M., 1049, 1051, 1107, 1117
Lemon, F.R., 306

Leo, T.F., 1270
Leon, R.G., 1039
Leopardi, E.A., 1158
Leslie, G.L., 809
Lester, C.W., 214
Levin, I., 995
Levine, N.D., 978
Levine, V.E., 1463
Levinson, R.A., 897
Levy, J.E., 1078
Levy, W.J., 1368
Lewis, L.A., 1267
Librik, L., 1345
Liebow, I.M., 1279
Lifschitz, M., 917
Lincoln, D.F., 23
Lindeman, R.D., 123
Lindert, M.C., 660A
Littman, B., 1174
Livermore, A.R., 1398
Lizotte, A., 1211
Lobban, M.D., 1347
Long, E.R., 830, 834, 837
Longman, D.P., 126
Loree, D.R., 52
Lorimer, F., 93
Lorincz, A.B., 1066
Lossing, E.H., 693
Loughlin, B.W., 570, 1153
Lowry, R.B., 1203
Lutwak, L., 149

Mabry, D.E., 1063
McAlister, R., 785
McCammon, C.S., 482, 930, 1147
McCaskill, J.C., 1024
McClellan, E., 1126
McClellan, T.E., 1448
McClenachan, H.M., 28
McCollum, R.W., 712
McDermott, W., 300, 538
McDonald, B.S., 1291, 1467
Macdonald, R.A., 694
McDougall, J.B., 859
McGee, M.D., 1222, 1309
McGibony, J.R., 471, 474, 747, 849
McHenry, H., 215
McKenzie, F.A., 1022
Mackinnon, A.G., 963
MacLean, C.J., 1156
McMahon, L.J., 1019
McMichael, E.V., 211
McMinimy, D.J., 853

McNeilly, M.M., 307
McNutt, C.W., 1318
Maddy, K.T., 659
Maher, S.J., 813
Mahon, W.A., 763
Malarkey, H.F., 1454
Mandell, G.L., 666, 1326
Mantling, G., 972
Marchand, J.F., 656
Marquis, J.R., 1295, 1304
Marshall, L.R., 271
Martens, E.G., 598
Martin, A.R., 957
Martin, M., 1033
Massey, W.C., 2
Matas, M., 919
Mathews, P.W., 29
Mathews, W.H., 938
Matthews, W., 790, 791, 793
Matwichuk, Z., 912
Maxted, W.R., 776
Mayberry, R.H., 123
Mayhall, J.T., 1428, 1439
Maynard, J.E., 703, 711, 970, 1277, 1476
Mays, T.J., 792
Mead, P.A., 898
Means, H.J., 161
Meehan, J.P., 1350
Meek, E.G., 230
Meerovitch, E., 935
Mehta, J.D., 217, 217A
Meltzer, H.L., 984
Melvin, D.M., 689
Menegaz-Bock, R.M., 1403
Merrill, R.G., 1417
Michael, J.M., 638
Michael, L.F., 262
Mickelson, N.I., 1044
Mico, P.R., 556, 557, 573
Middleton, A.E., 446
Milan, F.A., 145, 147
Miles, J.E., 1102
Millar, J., 1282
Millard, T.F., 242
Miller, D.C., 1271
Miller, J.R., 1187
Miller, M., 1320, 1327
Miller, M.J., 938, 982
Miller, S.I., 1079
Mills, L.F., 660
Molonhon, K.T., 1383
Monahan, G.F., 1340

Montgomery, L.G., 819, 824
Montross, H.E., 1231
Moodie, R.L., 159, 160, 164, 166, 167, 172, 1371
Moody, C.I., 87
Moody, C.S., 37
Moore, A., 349
Moore, D.F., 938
Moore, J.G., 218
Moore, M., 972
Moore, M.S., 771
Moore, P.E., 104, 355, 359, 476, 507, 514, 844, 900
Moore, P.H., 983
Moorman, L.J., 65, 293
Morgan, M., 1376
Morley, L.A., 508
Morris, D.H., 1429, 1440
Morris, J.W., 1244
Morse, D., 198
Moses, 21
Mountain, J.W., 459
Mouratoff, G.J., 1334
Mulvaney, W.P., 207
Mundt, R., 468
Murphy, J.A., 442, 804
Murray, W.W., 608
Muschenheim, C., 319
Muskakoo, V.E., 321
Myers, J.A., 854
Myers, S.E., 1418

Nagler, F.P., 727
Nasi, J.H., 1430
Neave, J.L., 32, 41
Neel, J.V., 333
Nelms, J.D., 142
Nelson, C.T., 1394
Nelson, L.G., 1099
Neter, E., 783
Neumann, H.W., 201
Newman, M.T., 116, 120
Newton, E.E., 445
Newton, J.B., 1223
Newton, J.K., 766
Nichols, J.V.V., 1358
Nicholson, M.W., 908
Nigg, C., 764
Niswander, J.D., 1156, 1157, 1188, 1191, 1196, 1197, 1328
Noble, T.B., 1266
Nowak, J., 588, 639

O'Brien, W.M., 1171, 1233, 1236, 1240, 1241, 1253
O'Connell, D.J., 1302
Old, H.N., 500
Omran, R., 918
Opler, M.E., 1084
Oren, J., 698
Orr, H., 931
Orton, G.T., 796
Osborne, M.D., 1342
Overfield, M., 785
Owen, W.B., 684

Page, I.H., 1267
Paine, A.L., 840, 912
Painter, S.L., 1287
Palmer, C.E., 850, 852, 922
Palmer, E.P., 999, 1001
Palmer, H.E., 153–156
Pandola, G., 660A
Pankow, G., 1032
Parfitt, G.J., 1408
Parker, A.C., 1023
Parker, L., 530
Parker, M.T., 776
Parks, G., 631
Parks, J.H., 1316
Parnell, I.N., 685
Parr, E.I., 842, 971
Parran, T., 510
Parrish, J., 10
Partridge, R.A., 783
Pasinsky, S.H., 1213
Patrie, L.E., 558
Paul, F.L., 875
Paul, J.R., 1263
Pauls, F.P., 501, 673
Payne, W., 132
Paynter, L.E., 827
Peart, A.F.W., 727
Perez, L.K., Jr., 546
Perking, G.B., 1212
Perkins, A.E., 1082
Perlman, L.V., 773, 775, 777
Perrott, G. St. J., 517
Perry, T.L., 1173, 1175
Peters, J.P., 572
Petersen, K., 1335
Petrakis, N.L., 1383, 1386
Pett, L.B., 107
Pfister, O., 1083
Philip, C.B., 960, 964

Philip, R.N., 704, 757, 899, 968, 970
Phillips, A.J., 1002, 1003
Phillips, F.J., 901, 906
Pijoan, M., 482, 780, 848, 1205, 1461
Pincock, T.A., 1060
Pitcher, Z., 435
Pitney, E.H., 92, 1392
Pollitzer, W.S., 1284
Poole, J.B., 985, 986, 988
Porter, M.E., 907
Porter, V.S., 1283
Portney, G.L., 640, 1365, 1369
Porvaznik, J., 327
Posers, D.K., 753
Posey, W.C., 731, 732
Post, P.W., 219
Pournelle, A.T., 1158
Pousma, R.H., 927
Powers, D.K., 755
Price, G.E., 1237–1239, 1243
Price, W.A., 103, 460, 655, 1389, 1390
Procter, H.A., 623
Prosnitz, L.R., 666, 1326
Prouty, M., 1281
Pusey, W.A., 724

Quie, P.Q., 779
Quiring, D.P., 136

Rabeau, E.S., 583, 642
Rabin, D.L., 1189
Rabkin, S., 188, 189
Radbill, S.X., 475
Rader, V., 681
Ranke, K., 238
Rankin, L.S., 1122
Rath, O.J.S., 590
Raup, M., 533
Rausch, R.L., 943–947, 980, 991
Reaud, A., 642
Reichenbach, D., 329
Reifel, A., 860
Reinhard, K.R., 695, 696, 713–716, 761
Reinstein, C.R., 770
Rentiers, R.L., 931
Renwick, D.H.G., 1203
Resnick, L., 1215
Rice, C.E., 182
Rice, P.F., 443
Richards, W.G., 820

Richey, D.F., 1480
Rider, A.S., 839
Rihan, H.Y., 174
Riley, H.D., Jr., 1198, 1214, 1216
Rimoin, D.L., 1329, 1330, 1336
Ringle, O.F., 821
Ritchie, W.A., 175, 187, 194
Roberts, B.J., 573
Robertson, G.G., 1103
Robinson, C.L.N., 925
Robinson, H.S., 1234, 1238, 1239, 1243, 1246
Rodahl, K., 1337, 1339
Rogers, A.G., 1303
Rogers, B.H.G., 1307
Romanowsky, 16
Romanowsky, P., 74
Romig, J.H., 75
Rosa, F., 1215
Rose, T.H., 478
Roseberg, J., 1117
Rosenbaum, L.J., 1366, 1367, 1370
Ross, C.A., 908
Ross, E.L., 840
Rothrock, J.L., 1144
Rubensten, A., 643
Rush, B., 9
Rymer, S., 644

Saeger, A.L., Jr., 1154
Saiki, J.H., 1329, 1330, 1343
St. Childs, J.R., 977
St. Hoyme, L.E., 199, 220
Saliba, G., 969
Salisbury, L.H., 298
Salsbury, C.G., 277, 288, 294, 453, 873, 1005, 1006, 1008
Sampliner, J.E., 1302
Sandison, A.T., 210
Saunders, A.L., 1004
Saunders, L.G., 686
Savard, R.J., 1069
Saylor, R.M., 842, 971
Schaefer, O., 71, 303, 1056, 1464
Schlafman, I.H., 645
Schmitt, N., 1473, 1474
Schneider, R.G., 1289
Schnur, L., 472
Schoolcraft, H.R., 17, 717
Schuck, C., 119, 121, 127
Schwartz, J.R., 1364
Schwartzmann, J.R., 1185

Scott, E.M., 122, 128, 129, 1162, 1163, 1165, 1166, 1168, 1283, 1285, 1334
Sedlacek, B., 848
Sega, S., 1181
Seid, S.E., 683
Seltzer, R.A., 574
Senter, R.G., 1254
Shands, J.R., Jr., 184
Shapiro, B.L., 1200
Shapiro, H.E., 214
Shattuck, G.C., 929
Shaw, J.R., 512, 518
Shaw, M.M., 134
Shaw, W.F., 44
Sheehan, J.F., 1017
Sherwood, N.P., 764
Ship, I.I., 1432, 1433
Shook, D.C., 646
Shoop, J.D., 926
Shufeldt, R.W., 1109
Sievers, M.L., 324, 902, 974, 1011, 1070, 1278, 1280, 1295, 1304, 1308
Silcott, M.E., 547
Silva, J.A., 903
Simes, A.B., 827, 858
Simmet, R., 539
Simmons, J.J., 513
Simmons, J.S., 49
Simmons, W.H., 1361
Simon, J.R., 684
Simpson, J.K., 1133
Sinclair, H.M., 108
Siniscal, A.A., 748
Sirkin, J., 1180
Sloan, R.P., 456
Slobodin, R., 1098
Slotnick, H.E., 298
Smart, C., 226
Smith, J.E., 746
Smith, R.L., 1006, 1007, 1269
Snidecor, J.C., 1106
Sniffen, M.K., 88
Snyder, R.G., 197
Solman, V.E.F., 949
Sparger, C.F., 1262, 1310, 1481, 1483
Spector, B.K., 670
Spicer, R.B., 292
Spitzer, A., 1028
Spruce, G.B., Jr., 1410
Stage, T.B., 1101

Stallings, W.S., Jr., 191
Stanfield, F.S., 950
Stanley, H.R., 1419
Stearn, A.E., 725
Stearn, E.A., 725
Steele, J.P., 202, 205
Stefansson, V., 117, 1010
Steggerda, M., 102, 1391, 1399
Stein, J.H., 1321
Stein, S.C., 876
Steinmetz, N., 611, 624
Sterling, E.B., 1141
Stevenson, A.H., 548, 601
Stewart, D.A., 828, 835
Stewart, J.L., 1108
Stewart, O., 1121
Stewart, T.D., 221, 1183, 1184
Sticker, G., 47
Stirling, M.W., 1478
Stoll, A.M., 1350
Stone, E., 48, 50, 264
Stone, E.L., 457, 808
Strandskov, H.H., 95
Stratton, T., 223
Straus, R., 1272, 1274
Streeper, R.B., 1273
Sturtevant, C., 3
Suckley, G., 22
Sumpter, G., 602
Swan, R., 81
Sweatman, G.K., 981

Talcott, M.I., 119, 121
Taugher, P.J., 660A
Taylor, H.C., 883, 890
Taylor, M.S., 503
Tchang, S., 939
Telford, C.W., 1111
Tello, J.C., 168
Templin, D., 923
Tepper, D.J., 1383
Terry, E., 503
Therrier, E., 866
Thomas, G.W., 561, 882, 909, 1012, 1150
Thomas, R.E., 653
Thomas, W.D.S., 1159
Thomassen á Thuersink, E.J., 13
Thompson, R.R., 82
Thompson, S., 591
Thorne, B., 1076
Thorworth, J.F., 30

Thwaites, R.G., 34, 35
Thygeson, P., 744, 753, 1351–1355, 1363
Tiber, B.M., 473, 483, 549
Tillim, S.J., 272, 273, 741
Tirador, D.F., 959
Titterington, P.E., 187
Tobey, J.A., 447
Toner, J.M., 25, 26
Toone, W.M., 836
Torrey, E.F., 1014
Townsend, J.G., 55, 278, 283, 375, 459, 461, 462, 745, 845–847
Towsley, A.C., 612
Tranter, C.L., 1091
Treon, F., 232, 699, 1129
Tretsven, V.E., 1186
Trowbridge, N., 1119
Truemen, G.E., 1246
Turner, C.G., 1457
Twinn, C.R., 488
Tyler, C.W., Jr., 1154
Tyler, I., 591

Uhrich, R.B., 647
Upadhyay, Y.N., 668
Updyke, E.L., 771
Urbanich, E.M., 1376
Urquhart, J.A., 53

Vall-Spinosa, A., 1071
Van Arsdell, W., 729
Van der Veer, J.B., Jr., 784
Van Duzen, J., 1470
Van Duzen, J.L., 76
Van Hagen, G.E., 857
Van Rooyen, C.E., 691
Van Sandt, M., 503
Van Wart, A.F., 290
Vavich, M.G., 110
Vernier, R., 777
Vincentia, S., 550
Vivian, R.P., 106

Wagner, C.J., 582, 583
Wagner, M.G., 1174
Wakefield, E.G., 101
Waldron, M.M., 438
Waldron, M.P.D., 778
Walker, J.R., 800
Walkin, F., 281
Wall, J.J., 739, 740

Wallace, A.F., 1097
Wallace, H.M., 921
Wallach, E.E., 1155
Walsh, J.J., 1110
Walton, C.H.A., 831
Wannamaker, L.W., 775
Ward, K.A., 69
Warner, H.J., 737, 822
Warwick, O.H., 1002
Waskow, E., 1316
Watkins, J.H., 92
Watson, E.L., 464, 477
Wauneka, A.D., 562
Webb, C.H., 1396, 1400
Webb, D.W., 649
Webb, G.B., 191
Weiss, E.S., 872, 878
Wellman, K.F., 540
Wells, C., 206
Wenberg, B.G., 121, 127
West, J.T., 989
West, M.D., 517
Westley, R., 1346
Whaley, H.S., 910
Wheatley, W., 784
Wherrett, G.J., 349
White, C.B., 97
White, W.D., 1323
Whiteford, L.J., 563, 576
Whitney, W.F., 31
Whittaker, J.O., 1057, 1058
Wicks, E.O., 564
Wiens, A.A., 551
Wilcox, E.B., 1465
Wilkes, C., 14
Williams, C.D., 187
Williams, H.V., 40, 168, 176, 180
Williams, R.B., 781, 782, 886, 961, 962
Williamson, R.G., 1041
Williamson, T., 228
Willis, J.S., 314, 534, 1030, 1033
Wilson, C.S., 493, 504
Wilson, J.F., 1259, 1260
Wilson, M.R., 584
Wilt, J.C., 950
Winder, W., 15
Winkler, A.M., 1072
Winter, L.H., 904
Winters, S.R., 285
Wissler, C., 56, 274, 275, 279, 1143
Wolfe, C.B., 1466

Wolfgang, R.W., 985, 986, 994
Wolman, C., 1125
Woodruff, C.E., 234
Woods, O.T., 289
Woodville, L., 585
Woodward, 976
Woolf, C.M., 1167, 1170, 1176, 1190
Work, H., 448
Work, T.H., 951
Worley, J.F., 465
Wright, R.E., 1283
Wrigley, J., 920
Wuerffel, S., 130
Wurm, M., 1272, 1274
Wyman, L., 1076

Wythe, W.T., 24

Yarrow, H.C., 84, 233
Yearsley, E., 118
Yost, G., 1192
Young, H.A., 498
Young, R.W., 308
Yule, R.F., 59

Zaruba, F., 1228
Zeis, D.M., 524
Zillatus, M.G., 565
Zimmerman, R.A., 767
Zimmermann, B., 211
Zonis, R.D., 1384, 1387

SUBJECT INDEX*

Accidents, 31, 97, 259, 298, 315, 316, 324, 365, 373, 378, 490, 590, 594, 1208, 1482 (see also TRAUMA AND ACCIDENTS)
Achlorhydria, 1308
Addiction, 1063, 1066 (see also ALCOHOLISM AND ADDICTION)
Addison's disease, 1340
Ague (see INFECTIOUS AGENTS AND DISEASES)
Air ambulance, 561
Albinism, 235, 243, 245, 246, 1161, 1169, 1170, 1176, 1190
Alcoholism, 22, 223, 225, 304, 319, 365, 490, 996, 1082, 1311, 1322, 1474 (see also ALCOHOLISM AND ADDICTION)
ALCOHOLISM AND ADDICTION, 1045–1075 (see also Addiction; Alcoholism; Drug abuse; Drug therapy for alcoholism; Narcotics)

Allergies, 296, 380–385, 387–389, 391–394, 396, 398, 400, 402, 403, 405, 407, 408, 410, 412–424, 426–431, 433
Alopecia, 1230
Amebiasis, 617, 689, 934–939, 942 (see also Parasitic diseases)
Amenorrhea, 1342
Anemia, 1205, 1282, 1283, 1290, 1291
Anhidrotic ectodermal dysplasia, 1192
Ankylosing spondylitis, 1239, 1245, 1246, 1249
Annual reports (see STATISTICAL PUBLICATIONS AND ANNUAL REPORTS)
Appendicitis, 288
Arbovirus, 951
ARCHEOLOGICAL STUDIES AND PALEOPATHOLOGY, 158–221
Arthritis, 212, 223, 277, 288, 1171, 1172, 1231, 1234, 1237, 1238, 1245,

*Small cap entries refer to the section titles.

131

1247, 1252 (see also Rheumatoid arthritis; Osteoarthritis; Ankylosing spondylitis)

Ascariasis, 942

Assistants (see Nursing assistants)

Asthma, 11, 324, 1257, 1464 (see also DISEASES OF THE RESPIRATORY SYSTEM [CHRONIC])

Atherosclerosis, 68, 315, 324, 1266, 1269, 1316 (see also DISEASES OF THE CARDIOVASCULAR SYSTEM; Coronary artery disease; Peripheral vascular disease)

Atherosclerotic heart disease (see Coronary artery disease)

Autobiography (see HISTORICAL, BIOGRAPHICAL, AUTOBIOGRAPHICAL, AND PERSONAL NARRATIVES)

Autoimmune disorder, 1344

Autopsy, 305, 316, 325, 1327

Bacterial bronchitis and pneumonias, 761–763, 1223 (see also DISEASES OF THE RESPIRATORY SYSTEM [CHRONIC]; Pneumonia)

Bacterial infections, 761–788, 953–970 (see also INFECTIOUS AGENTS AND DISEASES)

Bacterial meningitis, 788

BCG vaccine, 842, 850–852, 855, 856, 858, 868, 871, 876, 877, 883, 890, 917

Beta-isobutyric aciduria, 1165

BIBLIOGRAPHIES, 1–6

Bifid uvula, 1200

Biliary tract disease (see Gallbladder disease)

Biography (see HISTORICAL, BIOGRAPHICAL, AUTOBIOGRAPHICAL, AND PERSONAL NARRATIVES)

Birth (see PREGNANCY, CHILDBIRTH, AND GYNECOLOGICAL CONDITIONS)

Birth defect (see Congenital malformations)

Birth weight, 1156, 1157

Blindness, 1361 (see also DISEASES OF THE EYE)

Blood diseases, 296, 380–385, 387–389, 391–394, 396, 398–400, 402, 403, 405, 407, 408, 410, 412–424, 426–431, 433 (see also DISEASES OF THE HEMATOPOIETIC SYSTEM)

Bone diseases, 161, 173, 866 (see also DISEASES OF THE MUSCULOSKELETAL SYSTEM)

Brain disorders (see DISEASES OF THE NERVOUS SYSTEM)

Breast diseases (see DISEASES OF THE INTEGUMENTARY SYSTEM)

Bronchiectasis, 1259, 1260

Bronchitis (see Bacterial bronchitis and pneumonias)

Brucella abortus (see Brucellosis)

Brucellosis, 970

Burns (see TRAUMA AND ACCIDENTS)

Cancer (see Neoplasms)

Carcinoma (see Neoplasms)

Carcinoma of the cervix, 1008, 1009, 1013, 1017, 1021 (see also Neoplasms)

Cardiovascular system diseases, 68, 296, 304, 380–385, 387–389, 391–394, 396, 398–400, 402, 403, 405, 407, 408, 410, 412–424, 426–431, 433, 1002, 1006, 1007 (see also DISEASES OF THE CARDIOVASCULAR SYSTEM)

Caries (see DENTAL STUDIES AND PROBLEMS)

Cataracts, 296, 380–385, 387–389, 391–394, 396, 398–400, 402, 403, 405, 407, 408, 410, 412–424, 426–431, 433

Central nervous system diseases (see DISEASES OF THE NERVOUS SYSTEM)

Central nervous system infections, 683, 698, 788

Cerebrovascular disease, 296, 380–385, 387–389, 391–394, 396, 398–400, 402, 403, 405, 407, 408, 410, 412–424, 426–431, 433, 1269, 1473

Chemotherapy for tuberculosis, 880, 889, 905, 907 (see also Tuberculosis)

Childbirth (see PREGNANCY, CHILDBIRTH, AND GYNECOLOGICAL CONDITIONS)

Child health, 149, 332, 475, 531, 592, 611, 613, 624, 643, 735, 744, 754, 763, 785, 805, 819, 822, 827, 834, 856, 910, 921, 957, 1031, 1042, 1056, 1099, 1100, 1281, 1392, 1430 (see also CHILD HEALTH AND DISEASES OF INFANCY)

CHILD HEALTH AND DISEASES OF IN-

FANCY, 1204–1225 (see also Diseases of infancy; Child health; Congenital malformations; Childhood tuberculosis)

Childhood tuberculosis, 922

Cholecystitis (see Gallbladder disease)

Cholera, 81, 648, 652

Cholesterol, 1267, 1280 (see also DISEASES OF THE CARDIOVASCULAR SYSTEM)

Chronic obstructive lung disease (see DISEASES OF THE RESPIRATORY SYSTEM)

Circulatory system diseases (see DISEASES OF THE CARDIOVASCULAR SYSTEM)

Cirrhosis, 324, 325, 329, 1311 (see also DISEASES OF THE DIGESTIVE SYSTEM)

Cleft lip and/or palate, 1186, 1196, 1200, 1202, 1203 (see also Congenital malformations)

Clinics, 497, 523, 901, 1222, 1367

CNS diseases (see DISEASES OF THE NERVOUS SYSTEM)

Coccidioidomycosis, 306, 659, 971, 974, 975

Cold, 139, 141, 143–148, 151 (see also UPPER AND LOWER RESPIRATORY INFECTIONS)

Color blindness, 1177

Community health workers, 598, 600, 614

Congenital deafness, 1190

Congenital ear defect, 1199

Congenital hip dislocation, 538, 1181, 1185, 1189

Congenital malformations, 169, 173, 177, 181, 204, 209, 214, 223, 235, 296, 304, 305, 316, 325, 329, 378, 380–385, 387–389, 391–394, 396, 398–400, 402, 403, 405, 407, 408, 410, 412–424, 426–431, 433, 538, 1006, 1007, 1161–1203, 1212, 1281, 1327, 1331, 1387, 1389, 1417, 1426, 1428, 1439, 1464, 1473 (see also Congenital deafness; Congenital ear defect; Congenital hip dislocation; CHILD HEALTH AND DISEASES OF INFANCY; Cleft lip and/or palate; Inborn errors of metabolism)

Congressional investigations, 339, 341–344, 346, 347, 360, 365–371 (see also HEALTH SURVEYS, CONGRESSIONAL INVESTIGATIONS, AND LEGISLATION)

Conjunctivitis, 232 (see also Trachoma; Phlyctenular kerato-conjunctivitis)

Consumption (see Tuberculosis)

Contraceptives, 1155

Coronary artery disease, 123, 292, 296, 305, 315, 316, 324, 329, 380–385, 387–389, 391–394, 396, 398–400, 402, 403, 405, 407, 408, 412–424, 426–431, 433, 538, 590, 594, 825, 1265, 1267–1273, 1275, 1277–1279, 1473 (see also Atherosclerosis; DISEASES OF THE CARDIOVASCULAR SYSTEM; Heart disease)

Crime, 1006, 1007, 1114, 1117, 1121, 1206, 1224

Cystic fibrosis, 1198

Deafness, 164, 1371, 1377, 1378 (see also DISEASES OF THE EAR)

Dental assistants (see Nursing assistants)

Dental caries (see DENTAL STUDIES AND PROBLEMS)

DENTAL STUDIES AND PROBLEMS, 1388–1460 (see also Teeth disorders; Periodontal disease)

Depression (see Psychotic and psychoneurotic disorders)

Diabetes mellitus, 123, 288, 296, 324, 325, 380–385, 388, 389, 391–394, 396, 398–400, 402, 403, 405, 407, 408, 410, 412–424, 426–431, 433, 574, 1264, 1279, 1308, 1312–1336, 1464, 1480

Diaphorase deficiency, 1166, 1168

Diarrhea (see Dysentery)

DIET, NUTRITION, AND GROWTH, 101–132 (see also MALNUTRITION AND VITAMIN DEFICIENCIES)

Digestive system diseases, 235, 245, 296, 378, 380–385, 387–389, 391–394, 396, 398–400, 402, 403, 405, 407, 408, 410, 412–424, 426–431, 433, 538, 666, 1002, 1006 (see also DISEASES OF THE DIGESTIVE SYSTEM)

Diphyllobothriasis, 993, 994

Diphyllobothrium latum (see Diphyllobothriasis)

Diseases, infectious (see INFECTIOUS AGENTS AND DISEASES)

Diseases of the blood (see DISEASES OF THE HEMATOPOIETIC SYSTEM)

Diseases of the breast (see DISEASES OF THE INTEGUMENTARY SYSTEM)

DISEASES OF THE CARDIOVASCULAR SYSTEM, 1263–1280 (see also Cardiovascular system diseases; Coronary artery disease; Atherosclerosis; Cholesterol; Hypertension; Peripheral vascular disease; Rheumatic fever; Rheumatic valvulitis; Cerebrovascular disease)

Diseases of the circulatory system (see DISEASES OF THE CARDIOVASCULAR SYSTEM)

DISEASES OF THE DIGESTIVE SYSTEM, 1293–1311 (see also Digestive system diseases; Gallbladder disease; Cirrhosis; Gastrointestinal diseases; Liver diseases; Peptic ulcer)

DISEASES OF THE EAR, 1371–1387 (see also Ear diseases; Deafness; Ear infections)

DISEASES OF THE ENDOCRINE SYSTEM, 1312–1345 (see also Endocrine system diseases; Thyroid disorders)

DISEASES OF THE EYE, 1351–1370 (see also Eye diseases; Blindness; Cataracts; Color blindness; Conjunctivitis; Phlyctenular kerato-conjunctivitis; Trachoma)

DISEASES OF THE HEMATOPOIETIC SYSTEM, 1281–1292 (see also Blood diseases; Hemoglobinopathy)

Diseases of Indians—not specified (see INDIAN HEALTH AND DISEASE—UNSPECIFIED)

Diseases of infancy, 296, 380–385, 387–389, 391–394, 396, 398–400, 402, 403, 405, 407, 408, 410, 412–424, 426–431, 433 (see also CHILD HEALTH AND DISEASES OF INFANCY)

DISEASES OF THE INTEGUMENTARY SYSTEM, 1226–1230 (see also Skin diseases)

DISEASES OF THE MUSCULOSKELETAL SYSTEM, 1231–1255 (see also Musculoskeletal system diseases; Bone diseases; Orthopedic problems; Osteoarthritis)

DISEASES OF THE NERVOUS SYSTEM, 1348–1350 (see also Nervous system diseases; Central nervous system infections)

DISEASES OF THE RESPIRATORY SYSTEM (CHRONIC), 1256–1262 (see also Asthma; UPPER AND LOWER RESPIRATORY INFECTIONS; Respiratory diseases; Respiratory viral infections; Bacterial bronchitis and pneumonias; Cold; Pneumonia; Pulmonary diseases)

Diseases of the skin (see DISEASES OF THE INTEGUMENTARY SYSTEM)

DISEASES OF THE UROGENITAL SYSTEM, 1346–1347 (see also Genitourinary diseases; Renal diseases; Nephritis)

DISEASES TRANSMITTED FROM ANIMALS, ANIMAL PRODUCTS, OR SOIL TO MAN, 943–994

DISEASES TRANSMITTED FROM MAN TO MAN, 691–942

Drug abuse, 1091 (see also ALCOHOLISM AND ADDICTION)

Drug prophylaxis (see Chemotherapy for tuberculosis)

Drugs, 593, 597, 620, 632

Drug therapy for alcoholism, 1069, 1971 (see also ALCOHOLISM AND ADDICTION)

Dubin-Johnson syndrome, 1305

Dysentery, 224, 296, 380–385, 387–389, 391–394, 396, 398–400, 402, 403, 405, 407, 408, 410, 412–424, 426–431, 433, 575, 617, 643, 669, 671, 672, 679, 680, 783, 1473 (see also Gastrointestinal infections)

Ear diseases, 203, 296, 380–385, 387–389, 391–394, 396, 398–400, 402, 403, 405, 408, 410, 412–424, 426–431, 433, 528, 761 (see also DISEASES OF THE EAR)

Ear infections (see Upper respiratory infections; DISEASES OF THE EAR)

Echinococcosis, 980–991

Echinococcus granulosus and *multilocularis* (see Echinococcosis)

E. coli infections, 785–787 (see also Renal diseases)

Emphysema (see DISEASES OF THE RESPIRATORY SYSTEM [CHRONIC])

Empyema, 1258

Endocarditis, 1269

Endocrine system diseases, 296, 380–385, 387–389, 391–400, 402, 403, 405, 407, 408, 410, 412–424, 426–431, 433 (see also DISEASES OF THE ENDOCRINE SYSTEM)

Entamoeba histolytica (see Amebiasis)

Enteric infections (see Gastrointestinal infections)

Enteroviruses, 713, 715

ENVIRONMENTAL HEALTH, 152–157 (see also GENERAL HEALTH PROGRAMS AND SERVICES; Healthy environment)

Epidemiology, 566

Epilepsy, 223, 243, 245, 911, 1081, 1082, 1464

Eye diseases, 68, 182, 245, 287 (see also DISEASES OF THE EYE)

Family planning, 640, 642

Fluorosis, 1244

Focal epithelial hyperplasia, 1419

Fractures (see TRAUMA AND ACCIDENTS)

Fungal infections, 971–975

Gallbladder disease, 277, 296, 315, 325, 329, 380–385, 387–389, 391–394, 396, 398–400, 402, 403, 405, 407, 408, 410, 412–424, 426–431, 433, 1293–1302 (see also DISEASES OF THE DIGESTIVE SYSTEM)

Gastritis, 617

Gastroenteritis, 288, 296, 365, 380–385, 387–389, 391–394, 396, 398–400, 402, 403, 405, 407, 408, 410, 412–424, 426–431, 433, 590, 594, 617, 618, 1211 (see also Gastrointestinal infections)

Gastrointestinal diseases, 223, 243, 246, 259, 277, 291, 297, 316, 501, 835, 1293–1311 (see also DISEASES OF THE DIGESTIVE SYSTEM; Gastrointestinal infections)

Gastrointestinal infections, 323, 669–682 (see also Dysentery; Gastroenteritis; Gastrointestinal diseases)

GENERAL HEALTH PROGRAMS AND SERVICES, 435–647 (see also ENVIRONMENTAL HEALTH)

GENERAL TOPICS, 1–82

Genitourinary diseases, 378, 1007, 1366–1367 (see also DISEASES OF THE UROGENITAL SYSTEM)

Goiter, 124, 243, 245, 246, 654, 1337, 1339, 1344

Gout, 1171, 1172, 1464 (see also Inborn errors of metabolism)

Government and Indian health (see HEALTH PROGRAMS FOR INDIANS)

Growth and development, 131 (see also DIET, NUTRITION, AND GROWTH)

Gynecological conditions (see PREGNANCY, CHILDBIRTH, AND GYNECOLOGICAL CONDITIONS)

Hallerman-Streiff syndrome, 1195

Hand-Schüller-Christian disease, 1019

Health, mental (see MENTAL HEALTH AND PSYCHIATRIC DISORDERS)

Health aide (see Nursing Assistants)

Health auxiliaries (see Nursing assistants)

HEALTH PROGRAMS FOR INDIANS, 339–647 (see also Indian health programs)

Health services (see GENERAL HEALTH PROGRAMS AND SERVICES)

Health surveys, 341, 343–345, 347, 349, 351, 355, 358, 362, 363, 366, 505, 622, 1408 (see also HEALTH SURVEYS, CONGRESSIONAL INVESTIGATIONS, AND LEGISLATION)

HEALTH SURVEYS, CONGRESSIONAL INVESTIGATIONS, AND LEGISLATION, 339–371 (see also Health surveys; Legislation; Congressional investigations)

Healthy environment, 504, 580, 601, 615 (see also ENVIRONMENTAL HEALTH)

HEALTHY INDIVIDUALS, 83–157

Heart disease, 68 (see also Coronary artery disease)

Helminth infestations, 218, 684–690, 940–942, 980–994 (see also Intestinal parasites; Parasitic diseases)

Hematopoietic system disorders (see DISEASES OF THE HEMATOPOIETIC SYSTEM)

Hemoglobinopathy, 1284, 1285, 1288, 1289, 1292 (see also DISEASES OF THE HEMATOPOIETIC SYSTEM)

Hemophilia, 1287

Hepatitis, 296, 380–385, 387–389, 391–394, 396, 398–400, 402, 403,

405, 407, 408, 410, 412–424, 426–431, 433, 617, 708–712
Hermaphrodite, 1188
Histoplasmosis, 574, 659, 973
HISTORICAL, BIOGRAPHICAL, AUTOBIOGRAPHICAL, AND PERSONAL NARRATIVES, 7–82
Homicide, 1052, 1472 (see also TRAUMA AND ACCIDENTS)
Homosexuality, 1112
Hospitals, 446, 463, 464, 469, 474, 478, 523, 544, 584, 863, 881
Hydatid disease (see Echinococcosis)
Hygiene, 439, 475, 1022–1044
Hyperprolinaemia, 1175
Hypertension, 123, 124, 296, 324, 380–385, 387–389, 391–394, 396, 398–400, 402, 403, 405, 407, 408, 410, 412–424, 426–431, 433, 1264, 1268, 1269, 1275, 1278, 1326, 1464 (see also DISEASES OF THE CARDIOVASCULAR SYSTEM)
Hypertensive heart disease (see Hypertension)
Hypnosis, 1124
Hypothyroidism, 1338, 1343

Impetigo, 778 (see also DISEASES OF THE INTEGUMENTARY SYSTEM)
Inborn errors of metabolism, 1161–1176, 1285, 1287–1290, 1292, 1305
Incest, 1113
INDIAN HEALTH AND DISEASE—UNSPECIFIED, 158–338, 1002
Indian health programs, 55, 79, 291, 294, 300, 304, 309, 312, 313, 1402, 1404–1406, 1409, 1411, 1412, 1414, 1415, 1420, 1421, 1425, 1431, 1436, 1437, 1442, 1446, 1449, 1451, 1452, 1456, 1458–1460 (see also HEALTH PROGRAMS FOR INDIANS)
Infanticide, 1206
Infant mortality, 1200, 1204, 1209, 1215, 1217, 1218, 1220, 1225 (see also CHILD HEALTH AND DISEASES OF INFANCY)
INFECTIOUS AGENTS AND DISEASES, 648–994 (see also Infectious diseases; Bacterial infections; Central nervous system infections; Fungal infections; Gastrointestinal infections; Viral infections; Staphylococcal infections; Streptococcal infections, glomerulonephritic; Streptococcal infections, rheumatic; Respiratory viral infections; Rickettsial infections
Infectious diseases, 10, 47, 49, 51, 79, 97, 231, 243, 287, 289, 296–298, 304, 305, 315, 316, 324, 365, 377, 378–385, 387–433, 538, 564, 567, 594, 1006, 1007, 1158, 1375, 1376, 1378–1380, 1382, 1384, 1388, 1407 (see also INFECTIOUS AGENTS AND DISEASES)
Infestations, helminth (see Helminth infestations)
Influenza, 94, 277, 699–705
Injuries (see TRAUMA AND ACCIDENTS)
Insanity (see Psychiatric disorders)
Insecticides, 152
Insurance, 525
Intestinal parasites, 232 (see also Helminth infestations)
Investigations, congressional (see HEALTH SURVEYS, CONGRESSIONAL INVESTIGATIONS, AND LEGISLATION)

Kartagener's syndrome, 1193
Kerato-conjunctivitis (see Phlyctenular kerato-conjunctivitis)
Kwashiorkor, 1466, 1469

Legislation, 340, 348, 352–354, 356, 357, 360, 361, 364 (see also HEALTH SURVEYS, CONGRESSIONAL INVESTIGATIONS, AND LEGISLATION)
Lipids (see DISEASES OF THE CARDIOVASCULAR SYSTEM)
Liver diseases, 296, 380–385, 387–389, 391–394, 396, 398–400, 402, 403, 405, 407, 408, 410, 412–424, 426–431, 433 (see also DISEASES OF THE DIGESTIVE SYSTEM)
Lower respiratory infections (see UPPER AND LOWER RESPIRATORY INFECTIONS)
Lupus erythematosus, 1479

Malaria, 27, 68, 243, 245, 246, 652, 720, 976–979
Malformations, congenital (see Congenital malformations)
MALNUTRITION AND VITAMIN DEFICIENCIES, 1461–1470 (see also Vitamin deficiencies; Vitamin C deficiency; DIET, NUTRITION, AND GROWTH)

Malocclusion (see DENTAL STUDIES AND PROBLEMS)

Man to man transmission of disease (see DISEASES TRANSMITTED FROM MAN TO MAN)

Maternal mortality, 1141, 1152, 1159

Measles, 94, 240, 243, 245, 246, 296, 297, 380–385, 387–389, 391–394, 396, 398–400, 402, 403, 405, 407, 408, 410, 412–424, 426–431, 433, 522, 648, 652, 720, 722, 727–729

Medical school, 1043, 1482

Meningitis, 296, 380–385, 387–389, 391–394, 396, 398–400, 402, 403, 405, 407, 408, 410, 412–424, 426–431, 433, 683, 698, 788, 916, 957

Mental disorders, 296, 319, 378, 380–385, 387–389, 391–394, 396, 398–400, 402, 403, 405, 407, 408, 410, 412–414, 426–431, 433 (see also MENTAL HEALTH AND PSYCHIATRIC DISORDERS)

MENTAL HEALTH AND PSYCHIATRIC DISORDERS, 336, 365, 1022–1125 (see also Psychiatric disorders; Mental disorders)

Metabolism, 134–136, 138, 141, 143, 145–149 (see also PHYSIOLOGY AND METABOLISM)

Methemoglobinemia, 1162, 1163, 1165, 1166, 1168

Midwife (see PREGNANCY, CHILDBIRTH, AND GYNECOLOGICAL CONDITIONS)

Mongolism, 1179, 1180

Mucocele, 1020

Muscle diseases (see DISEASES OF THE MUSCULOSKELETAL SYSTEM)

Musculoskeletal system diseases, 296, 380–385, 387–389, 391–394, 396, 398–400, 402, 403, 405, 407, 408, 410, 412–424, 426–431, 433 (see also DISEASES OF THE MUSCULOSKELETAL SYSTEM)

Mycobacterium tuberculosis (see Tuberculosis)

Myeloma, 175

Myocardial infarction (see Coronary artery disease)

Narcotics, 619 (see also ALCOHOLISM AND ADDICTION)

Narratives (see HISTORICAL, BIOGRAPHICAL, AUTOBIOGRAPHICAL, AND PERSONAL NARRATIVES)

Neoplasms, 68, 123, 211, 288, 296, 304, 305, 315, 316, 324, 329, 378, 380–385, 387–389, 391–394, 396, 398–400, 402, 403, 405, 407, 408, 410, 412–424, 426–431, 433, 590, 594, 825, 995–1021, 1293, 1295, 1304, 1316, 1464, 1473 (see also Carcinoma of the cervix)

Nephritis, 1278 (see also Nephritogenic streptococci; DISEASES OF THE UROGENITAL SYSTEM)

Nephritogenic streptococci, 769–777 (see also Nephritis; Renal diseases)

Nervous system diseases, 296, 380–385, 387, 389, 394, 396, 398–400, 402, 403, 405, 407, 408, 410, 412–424, 426–431, 433, 898, 911, 1002, 1007 (see also DISEASES OF THE NERVOUS SYSTEM)

Neural arch defect, 1183, 1184

Neurological diseases (see DISEASES OF THE NERVOUS SYSTEM)

Neuropathy, 1326

Nursing, 454, 479, 483, 524, 532, 543, 550, 551, 565, 576, 589, 605, 620, 630

Nursing assistants, 542, 569, 570, 638, 646, 1422, 1423, 1434, 1435, 1445, 1448

Nutrition, 101–132, 289, 365, 533, 1390, 1398, 1401, 1433, 1461–1470

Nutritional deficiency (see MALNUTRITION AND VITAMIN DEFICIENCIES)

Obesity, 1480

Obstetrics (see PREGNANCY, CHILDBIRTH, AND GYNECOLOGICAL CONDITIONS)

Occupational therapy, 832

Oculomandibulodyscephaly, 1195

Orthopedic problems, 1232 (see also DISEASES OF THE MUSCULOSKELETAL SYSTEM)

Osteitis fibrosa, 170

Osteoarthritis, 200, 1251 (see also DISEASES OF THE MUSCULOSKELETAL SYSTEM)

Osteomyelitis, 190

Otitis media, 296, 380–385, 387–389, 391–394, 396, 398–400, 402, 403, 405, 407, 408, 410, 412–424, 426–

431, 433, 1375, 1376, 1378–1380, 1382, 1384

Paleopathology (see Archeological studies and paleopathology)
Paralysis (see Diseases of the nervous system)
Parasitic diseases, 296, 380–385, 387–389, 391–394, 396, 398–400, 402, 403, 405, 407, 408, 410, 412–424, 426–431, 433, 670, 676, 940, 941, 1322 (see also Amebiasis; Helminth infestations)
Pasteurella pestis (see Plague)
Pasteurella tularensis (see Tularemia)
Pathology, 133
Pediatric problems (see Child health and diseases of infancy)
Pentosuria, 1173
Peptic ulcer, 296, 324, 380–385, 387–389, 391–394, 396, 398–400, 402, 403, 405, 407, 408, 410, 412–424, 426–431, 433, 1304, 1306 (see also Diseases of the digestive system)
Periodontal disease, 1388, 1407, 1430 (see also Dental studies and problems)
Peripheral vascular disease, 1327 (see also Atherosclerosis; Diseases of the cardiovascular system)
Pernicious anemia, 31, 1286
Personal narratives (see Historical, biographical, autobiographical, and personal narratives)
Phenylketonuria, 1174
Phlyctenular kerato - conjunctivitis, 1351–1357
Photodermatitis, 1229
Physical fitness, 140, 150
Physical therapy, 608
Physiology, 135, 138–148, 151 (see also Physiology and metabolism)
Physiology and metabolism, 133–151 (see also Metabolism; Physiology)
Piebaldness, 1190
Plague, 40, 953–959
Pneumonia, 97, 224, 259, 277, 288, 291, 297, 522, 590, 594, 613, 618, 825, 1208, 1473 (see also Upper and lower respiratory infections; Bacterial bronchitis and pneumonias;

Diseases of the respiratory system)
Polio, 692–697
Portal hypertension, 1309
Pregnancy, 64, 124, 296, 306, 309, 378, 380–385, 387–389, 391–394, 396, 398–400, 402, 403, 405, 407, 408, 410, 412–424, 426–431, 433, 479, 590, 618, 1002, 1126–1160, 1464 (see also Pregnancy, childbirth, and gynecological conditions)
Pregnancy, childbirth, and gynecological conditions, 1126–1160 (see also Pregnancy)
Programs for Indians (see Health programs for indians)
Protozoal infestations (see Amebiasis; Malaria)
Psittacosis, 950
Psoriasis, 1228
Psychiatric disorders, 298, 1080–1103, 1213 (see also Mental health and psychiatric disorders)
Psychological testing, 1111, 1115, 1119, 1122
Psychoneurotic disorders (see Psychotic and psychoneurotic disorders)
Psychosomatic disorders, 1464
Psychotherapy, 1083, 1087, 1093, 1094, 1125
Psychotic and psychoneurotic disorders, 318, 1080–1103
Pterygium, 1365, 1369
Puberty, 1128
Pulmonary diseases, 1256 (see also Diseases of the respiratory system)
Pyelonephritis (see E. coli infections; Diseases of the urogenital system)
Pyorrhea (see Periodontal disease)

Q fever, 952

Rabies, 949
Radioactivity, 153–156
Radiology, 588, 871, 923, 939, 1244
Renal diseases, 296, 380–385, 387–389, 391–394, 396, 398–400, 402,

403, 405, 407, 408, 410, 412–424, 426–431, 433, 891, 920, 1326, 1346, 1347 (see also Nephritogenic streptococci; *E. coli* infections; DISEASES OF THE UROGENITAL SYSTEM)
Renal stones, 207
Reports, annual (see STATISTICAL PUBLICATIONS AND ANNUAL REPORTS)
Respiratory diseases, 223, 235, 246, 296, 316, 323, 380–385, 387–389, 391–394, 396, 398–400, 402, 403, 405, 407, 408, 410, 412–424, 426–431, 433, 667, 1002, 1006, 1007 (see also DISEASES OF THE RESPIRATORY SYSTEM [CHRONIC])
Respiratory viral infections, 706, 707 (see also DISEASES OF THE RESPIRATORY SYSTEM [CHRONIC])
Rheumatic fever, 296, 380–385, 387–389, 391–394, 396, 398–400, 402, 403, 405, 407, 408, 410, 412–424, 426–431, 433, 768, 1263, 1268, 1269, 1464
Rheumatic heart disease (see Rheumatic fever; Rheumatic valvulitis)
Rheumatic valvulitis, 296, 380–385, 387–389, 391–394, 396, 398–400, 402, 403, 405, 407, 408, 410, 412–424, 426–431, 433 (see also DISEASES OF THE CARDIOVASCULAR SYSTEM)
Rheumatism, 35 (see also Arthritis)
Rheumatoid arthritis, 1233, 1235, 1236, 1240–1243, 1245, 1248, 1250, 1253, 1255
Rickettsial infections, 952

Salmonella-shigella infections, 658, 679, 780–784 (see also Shigellosis)
Salmonellosis (see Salmonella-shigella infections)
Sanitation, 436–441, 479, 480, 500, 508, 511, 515, 520, 530, 541, 546, 548, 554, 555, 559, 586, 610, 615, 617, 641, 643
Scarlet fever (see Rheumatic fever)
Screening tests, 558, 574
Scrofula (see Tuberculosis)
Scurvy (see Vitamin C deficiency)
Selective service, 471
Services for Indians (see GENERAL HEALTH PROGRAMS AND SERVICES)

Sheehan's syndrome, 1341
Shigellosis, 784 (see Salmonella-shigella infections)
Skeletal system diseases (see DISEASES OF THE MUSCULOSKELETAL SYSTEM)
Skin diseases, 296, 380–385, 387–389, 391–394, 396, 398–400, 402, 403, 405, 407, 408, 410, 412–424, 426–431, 433, 775, 866, 1192 (see also DISEASES OF THE INTEGUMENTARY SYSTEM)
Smallpox, 22, 27, 81, 94, 225, 231, 237, 239, 240, 243, 245, 533, 572, 648, 652, 654, 717–726
Smoking, 1070
Snakebite, 1478, 1483
Social work, 547, 591, 603, 613
Spondylitis, 1258
Spondylosis, 1254
Sporotrichosis, 972
Staphylococcal infections, 778, 779
STATISTICAL PUBLICATIONS AND ANNUAL REPORTS, 372–433
Statistics, 560 (see also STATISTICAL PUBLICATIONS AND ANNUAL REPORTS; VITAL STATISTICS)
Streptococcal infections, glomerulonephritic, 769–777
Streptococcal infections, rheumatic, 764–768
Stroke, 123
STUDIES ON HEALTHY INDIVIDUALS, 83–157
Stuttering, 1104–1108
Surgery, 42, 48, 160, 926, 1477
Surgery for tuberculosis, 814, 894, 908, 912
Surveys (see HEALTH SURVEYS, CONGRESSIONAL INVESTIGATIONS, AND LEGISLATION)
Syphilis, 27, 168, 176, 178–180, 183, 184, 225, 240, 263, 490, 574, 650, 794, 927–933, 1348 (see also Venereal disease)

Teeth disorders, 162, 163, 165–167, 171, 172, 174, 188, 189, 197, 212, 217, 217A, 459, 855, 1009, 1182, 1194, 1322, 1475 (see also DENTAL STUDIES AND PROBLEMS)
Teratology (see Congenital malformations)

Thyroid disorders, 296, 380–385, 387–389, 391–394, 396, 398–400, 402, 403, 405, 407, 408, 410, 412–424, 426–431, 433, 1337–1339, 1343–1345 (see also DISEASES OF THE ENDOCRINE SYSTEM)
Thyrotoxicosis, 1344
Toxemia, 1152
Trachoma, 97, 245, 259, 277, 288, 291, 292, 297, 318, 319, 449, 522, 526, 617, 635, 654, 730–760, 996
Transvestite, 1178
Trauma, 161, 193, 228, 277, 296, 304, 373, 380–385, 387–389, 391–394, 396, 398–400, 402, 403, 405, 407, 408, 410, 412–424, 426–431, 433, 652, 825, 1224, 1262, 1309, 1464 (see also TRAUMA AND ACCIDENTS)
TRAUMA AND ACCIDENTS, 1471–1476 (see also Accidents; Trauma; Homicide)
Treponema pallidum (see Syphilis)
Trichinella spiralis (see Trichinosis)
Trichinosis, 992
Trichobezoar, 1307
Tuberculin skin test, 817, 895, 897, 917, 924,
Tuberculosis, 11, 14, 16, 22, 35, 97, 159, 191, 194, 198, 223–225, 228, 232, 240, 243, 245, 246, 259, 261, 287, 289, 292, 296–298, 300, 304–306, 309, 323, 325, 329, 359, 365, 380–385, 387–389, 391–394, 396, 398–400, 402, 403, 405, 407, 408, 410, 412–424, 426–431, 433, 494, 522, 526, 533, 572, 574, 575, 578, 590, 594, 618, 650, 654, 659, 789–926, 971, 996, 998, 1002, 1008, 1060, 1150, 1210, 1268, 1336, 1352, 1473 (see also Chemotherapy for tuberculosis; Childhood tuberculosis; Surgery for tuberculosis)
Tularemia, 658, 960–969
Twins, 1145
Typhoid fever, 654, 673
Typhus, 81

Ulcerative colitis, 1303
UPPER AND LOWER RESPIRATORY INFECTIONS, 662–668 (see also DISEASES OF THE RESPIRATORY SYSTEM [CHRONIC]; DISEASES OF THE EAR; Pneumonia)
Upper respiratory infections (see UPPER AND LOWER RESPIRATORY INFECTIONS)
Uric acid (see Gout)
Urogenital system diseases (see DISEASES OF THE UROGENITAL SYSTEM)
Uveitis, 1366

Venereal disease, 11, 22, 64, 97, 223, 235, 242, 243, 245, 287, 291, 297, 996, 1322 (see also Syphilis)
Violent deaths (see TRAUMA AND ACCIDENTS)
Viral infections, 691–760, 949–951
Viral meningitis, 698
VITAL STATISTICS, 83–100, 1187
Vitamin C deficiency, 848, 1461–1463, 1465, 1467
Vitamin deficiencies, 296, 380–385, 387–389, 391–394, 396, 398–400, 402, 403, 405, 407, 408, 410, 412–424, 426–431, 433 (see also MALNUTRITION AND VITAMIN DEFICIENCIES)

Whipple's disease, 660A

Zoonoses, 943–994

TRIBE INDEX

Acoma, 385, 420, 516, 750, 1271
Alabama-Coushatta, 1289, 1318
"Alaskan" Tribes Combined, 4, 42,
52, 58, 60, 63, 74, 76, 82, 88, 108,
109, 112, 115, 117, 122, 125, 128,
129, 137, 138, 140–148, 151–156,
186, 235, 247, 260, 287, 291, 298,
304, 312, 332, 347, 353, 355, 359,
440, 441, 460, 470, 501, 502, 504,
505, 508, 510, 511, 515, 520, 524,
527, 528, 530, 544, 552–555, 559,
560, 566, 571, 580, 582, 584, 598,
600, 623, 624, 637, 646, 655, 656,
657, 661–665, 673–678, 681, 687,
691–693, 695, 696, 703, 704, 708–
716, 727, 761, 781, 786–788, 798,
825, 838, 850, 851, 853, 856, 857,
863, 864, 868, 872, 875–881, 884,
886, 888–890, 893, 895, 898, 899,
901, 904–907, 909, 910, 913–916,
920, 944–946, 960–962, 964–970,
973, 980, 983, 985, 987, 989, 991,
993, 994, 1012, 1014–1016, 1047,
1049, 1055, 1056, 1096, 1123, 1133,
1149, 1162–1165, 1181, 1184, 1207–
1209, 1221, 1224, 1258–1260, 1264,
1277, 1283, 1285, 1290, 1337, 1339,
1347, 1350, 1354, 1356, 1357, 1359,
1362, 1372–1374, 1378, 1389, 1390,
1417, 1428, 1448, 1451, 1464, 1472,
1476
Apache (several tribes), 85, 86, 97,
123, 226, 227, 245, 249, 250, 296,
316, 319, 324, 329, 385, 389, 420,
428, 430, 516, 698, 728, 732, 743,
744, 751, 753, 754, 795, 799, 849,
883, 887, 932, 971, 974, 1011, 1021,
1052, 1064, 1070, 1081, 1084, 1114,
1120, 1121, 1149, 1155, 1156, 1157,
1195, 1264, 1270, 1275, 1278, 1279,
1295, 1296, 1302, 1304, 1308, 1312,
1314, 1346
Arapaho, 123, 380, 386, 430, 684, 747,
846, 850, 851, 856, 862, 864, 868,
876, 883, 890, 1042, 1149, 1174,
1212

141

Arikara, 382, 429, 690, 1111, 1139
Assiniboin, 124, 380, 532, 723, 811, 1149, 1157, 1186, 1335
Athabaskan (or Athapascan), 711, 1334

Bannock, 381, 414, 745, 1081
Blackfoot, 380, 445, 532, 697, 735, 747, 811, 849, 1009, 1028, 1081, 1135, 1171, 1172, 1186, 1233, 1236, 1241, 1245, 1251, 1253

Caddo, 123, 386, 430
"Canadian" Tribes Combined, 4, 15, 44, 53, 59, 62, 79, 100, 104, 105–107, 116–118, 136, 157, 267, 281, 302, 314, 320, 349, 376, 394, 457, 460, 488, 498, 509, 525, 552, 563, 576, 589, 590, 611, 644, 658, 685, 688, 705, 721, 738–740, 762, 763, 778, 805, 808, 810, 824, 826, 835, 840, 844, 858, 866, 882, 885, 891, 894, 900, 908, 911, 912, 919, 926, 931, 934, 935, 937, 938, 948, 949, 950, 952, 972, 981, 982, 984, 986, 988, 990, 992, 1003, 1004, 1030, 1033, 1050, 1051, 1060, 1085, 1102, 1108, 1150, 1152, 1159, 1175, 1184, 1187, 1194, 1203, 1211, 1219, 1220, 1223, 1229, 1232, 1237, 1238, 1246, 1255, 1256, 1282, 1303, 1338, 1340, 1357, 1379, 1395, 1424, 1457, 1464, 1468, 1473, 1474, 1479
Catawba, 386
Cayuse, 381, 422
Chehalis, 408
Chemehuevi, 324, 389, 428, 747, 1287, 1373
Cherokee, 20, 72, 90, 123, 204, 358, 386, 421, 430, 719, 807, 940, 942, 1081, 1149, 1156, 1157, 1198, 1296, 1321, 1344
Cheyenne, 235, 380, 386, 430, 532, 572, 702, 747, 757, 768, 820, 849, 1103, 1149, 1157, 1174, 1186
Chickasaw, 257, 386, 430, 832, 1264
Chinook, 22, 408, 1149
Chippewa, 35, 223, 380, 382, 424, 429, 449, 450, 532, 551, 572, 686, 690, 694, 769, 770–774, 776, 843, 846, 850, 851, 856, 862, 864, 868, 874, 876, 890, 1052, 1081, 1111,

1141, 1149, 1157, 1200, 1293, 1397, 1447
Choctaw, 116, 123, 386, 417, 430, 832, 1156, 1157, 1317, 1319
Clallam, 408, 1127
Clapsop (or Clatsop), 408
Cocopah, 324, 389, 428, 1278, 1296, 1325, 1333
Coeur d'Alene (or Skitswish), 381, 414
Comanche, 123, 239, 386, 430, 1149, 1155, 1157, 1226, 1320
Cree, 157, 811, 849, 1143, 1186, 1305, 1358, 1462, 1464
Creek, 72, 123, 386, 430, 1081, 1149, 1156, 1157
Crow, 246, 380, 516, 532, 702, 735, 747, 820, 849, 1103, 1149, 1156, 1157, 1186, 1271

Dakota, 231, 648
Delaware, 123, 386, 430

Flathead, 380, 532, 722, 747, 849, 1082, 1149, 1186

Goshute (or Gosiute), 1278
Gros Ventres, 124, 380, 532, 849, 1186

Haida, 1149, 1234, 1237, 1239, 1243, 1246
Havasupai, 389, 737, 1278
Hidatsa, 382, 429
Hoopa, 234, 389, 1278
Hopi, 76, 116, 245, 246, 249, 250, 293, 324, 389, 428, 737, 747, 753, 799, 874, 1011, 1032, 1070, 1071, 1147, 1149, 1155–1157, 1167, 1176, 1190, 1257, 1266, 1278, 1280, 1295, 1302, 1304, 1326, 1360, 1478
Hualapai, 324, 329, 389, 428, 1011, 1277, 1296, 1304
Hupa (or Hoopa), 802
Huron (or Wyandot), 797

Iowa, 386, 416, 430
Iroquois, 1054, 1149

Jemez, 420, 750, 1169

Kalispel (or Pend d'Oreilles), 381, 408

Karok, 30, 389
Kaw (or Kansa), 386, 430
Kickapoo, 123, 386, 416
Kiowa, 123, 239, 386, 430, 1157, 1198, 1226
Klamath, 422, 807, 1052
Kootenia, 380, 381, 414, 532
Kutenai, 1186

Laguna, 385, 420, 750, 1147, 1302, 1312
Lummi, 381, 408

Makah, 381, 408
Mandan, 382, 429, 724
Maricopa, 316, 324, 389, 428, 672, 679, 737, 1011, 1277, 1296, 1304, 1312
Menominee, 246, 382, 424, 802, 1046, 1081
Miami, 386, 430
Modoc, 381, 422
Mohave (or Mojave), 245, 316, 324, 329, 389, 428, 737, 795, 802, 1011, 1048, 1052, 1077, 1086, 1089, 1112, 1113, 1145, 1146, 1149, 1206, 1245, 1264, 1278, 1296, 1304, 1312, 1314, 1364, 1480
Mohawk, 1264
Munsee, 382, 424
Muskhogean, 1318

Navajo (or Navaho), 76, 80, 98, 102, 111, 116, 235, 245, 249, 250, 272, 277, 284, 288, 289, 291, 293, 297, 300, 306, 308, 309, 315, 316, 319, 324, 327, 329, 385, 389, 420, 423, 428, 453, 466, 472, 479, 482, 483, 512, 519, 521, 535, 538, 542, 556, 557, 569, 570, 573, 578, 591, 604, 625, 660, 666, 670, 671, 679, 683, 729, 732, 737, 750, 753, 754, 758, 760, 780, 795, 799, 848, 869, 892, 896, 917, 918, 927, 930, 954–959, 974, 996, 998, 1001, 1005, 1006, 1008, 1011, 1013, 1018, 1021, 1038, 1052, 1059, 1067–1071, 1074, 1076, 1078, 1079, 1081, 1083, 1087, 1090, 1099, 1121, 1125, 1141, 1147–1149, 1153, 1155–1157, 1160, 1168, 1178, 1189, 1195, 1199, 1210, 1213, 1217, 1257, 1261, 1264, 1265, 1267, 1269,

1272–1274, 1276, 1278, 1280, 1291, 1295–1297, 1301, 1302, 1304, 1308, 1310–1313, 1326, 1329, 1330, 1343, 1360, 1364, 1365, 1369, 1380, 1382, 1391, 1408, 1427, 1453, 1466, 1470, 1473–1476, 1478, 1482, 1483
Nez Perce, 87, 414, 747, 976
Nisqually (or Nisqualli), 408
Nooksack (or Nooksak), 408
Nootka, 1149

Omaha, 382, 418, 669, 690, 720, 941, 1046, 1052, 1149, 1463
Oneida, 246, 382, 424, 807, 1397
Onondaga, 225, 437
Opata, 245
Osage, 123, 386, 430, 1081
Oto-Missouri, 386, 430
Ottawa, 223, 382, 572, 1149

Paiute, 324, 389, 419, 422, 423, 516, 747, 754, 1081, 1149, 1155–1157, 1264, 1278, 1296, 1314
Papago, 96, 110, 116, 245, 291, 292, 296, 316, 319, 324, 329, 389, 428, 565, 616, 622, 737, 747, 753, 754, 799, 834, 971, 974, 1011, 1046, 1052, 1070, 1149, 1156, 1157, 1187, 1257, 1278, 1280, 1295, 1296, 1304, 1313, 1314, 1316, 1440, 1461
Passamaquoddy, 1330
Pawnee, 386, 430
Pend d'Orielle, 1186
Piegan, 380, 532
Pima, 95, 114, 245, 296, 316, 319, 324, 325, 329, 389, 428, 473, 652, 672, 679, 725, 737, 747, 752–754, 799, 846, 850, 851, 856, 862, 864, 868, 876, 883, 890, 971, 974, 1011, 1070, 1149, 1156, 1157, 1171, 1172, 1192, 1231, 1236, 1245, 1250, 1253, 1254, 1257, 1264, 1278–1280, 1294, 1296, 1298–1300, 1304, 1308, 1312–1314, 1316, 1320, 1327, 1387, 1403
Ponca, 123, 382, 386, 418, 430, 690
Potawatomi, 123, 382, 386, 416, 424, 430, 690, 1061, 1397
"Pueblo," 57, 92, 126, 135, 273, 385, 420, 516, 670, 737, 747, 750, 758, 765, 766, 799, 887, 1013, 1021, 1137, 1138, 1142, 1147, 1156,

1169, 1204, 1271, 1302, 1312, 1368, 1392, 1394
Puyallup, 408

Quapaw, 123, 386, 430
Quillayute (or Quileute), 381, 408
Quinaielt (or Quinault), 381, 408, 802

Salishan, 408, 722
San Juan, 1052, 1169
Sauk (Sak) and Fox, 382, 386, 415, 416, 430, 690
Seminole, 72, 91, 123, 345, 386, 413, 430, 579, 649, 951
Seneca, 116, 123, 240, 386, 430, 690, 1082, 1331A, 1340
Shawnee, 123, 386, 430, 897
Shoshone, 64, 380, 381, 389, 414, 419, 423, 747, 846, 850, 851, 856, 862, 864, 868, 876, 883, 890, 1205, 1212, 1278, 1296, 1314
Sioux, 119, 121, 127, 130, 149, 202, 205, 228, 232, 262, 380, 382, 418, 431, 451, 516, 532, 572, 651, 690, 699, 718, 735, 747, 794, 800, 802, 813, 846, 849–851, 856, 862, 864, 868, 869, 876, 883, 890, 933, 969, 994, 1052, 1057, 1058, 1066, 1081, 1111, 1129, 1140, 1141, 1149, 1156, 1157, 1186, 1193, 1257, 1293, 1306, 1307, 1335, 1432, 1477
Skagit, 381, 408
Skokomish, 408
Snohomish, 381
Snoqualmie (or Snoquamish), 381, 408

Spokan, 381, 408, 747
Stockbridge, 382, 424
Suquamish (or Squawmish), 408
Swinomish, 408

Tanoaen, 1157
Taos, 420, 760, 1278
Tonkawa, 123, 386, 430, 1317
Tonto, 1264

Umatilla, 381, 422, 747
Ute, 245, 324, 385, 389, 412, 423, 747, 795, 887, 1052, 1108, 1121, 1149, 1264, 1278, 1314

Walapai (or Hualapai), 245, 316, 737, 1264
Wallawalla, 381, 422
Warm Springs (or Tenino), 381, 422, 516
Washoe, 324, 389, 419, 1278
Wichita, 123, 386, 430
Winnebago, 18, 231, 382, 418, 424, 690, 807, 941, 1081, 1293

Yakima, 381, 422, 747, 784
Yavapai, 316, 324, 389, 679, 1011, 1278, 1296, 1304, 1312, 1316
Yuma, 33, 245, 324, 389, 679, 747, 1052, 1276, 1296, 1314
Yurok, 389

Zuni, 84, 116, 233, 235, 245, 246, 252, 253, 385, 420, 680, 737, 758, 932, 959, 1021, 1147, 1149, 1156, 1157, 1161, 1195, 1257, 1278, 1280, 1302

LINGUISTIC STOCK OF THE TRIBES
MENTIONED IN THE TRIBE INDEX*

"ALASKAN" (several tribes combined)
ALGONQUIN
 Arapaho
 Blackfoot (also Siouan)
 Cheyenne
 Chippewa (or Ojibway)
 Cree
 Delaware
 Gros Ventres
 Kickapoo
 Menominee
 Miami
 Munsee
 Ottawa
 Passamaquoddy
 Piegan
 Potawatomi
 Sauk (Sak) and Fox
 Shawnee
ATHAPASCAN
 Apache (several tribes)
 "Canadian Athapascan"
 Hupa (or Hoopa)
 Navajo (or Navaho)
CADDOAN
 Arikara
 Caddo
 Pawnee
 Wichita
"CANADIAN" (several tribes; many Athapascan)
CHIMAKUAN

*Arranged using the following aids:
  Wissler, C.: *American Indian*, 3rd ed, New York: Oxford U Press, 1938.
  Hodge, F.W.: *Handbook of American Indians North of Mexico*, Smithsonian Inst, Bur of Amer Ethnology, Bull No. 30, pts 1 and 2, Washington, DC, 1907, 1910.
  Swanton, J.R.: *The Indian Tribes of North America*, Smithsonian Inst, Bur of Amer Ethnology, Bull No. 145, Washington, DC, 1952.

Quillayute (or Quileute)
CHINOOKAN
Chinook
Clapsop (or Clatsop)
Flathead (some of them)
HOKAN (proposed name for Quora-
tean, Yuman, and some stocks not
mentioned here)
IROQUOIAN
Cherokee
Huron (or Wyandot)
Iroquois
Mohawk
Oneida
Onondaga
Seneca
KERESAN (see "PUEBLO")
Acoma
Laguna
KIOWA-TANOAN
Jemez
Kiowa
San Juan
Taos
KITUNAHAN
Kutenai
MAHICAN
Stockbridge
MUSKHOGEAN
Alabama-Coushatta
Chickasaw
Choctaw
Creek
Seminole
PIMAN (see UTO-AZTECAN)
Opata
Papago
Pima
"PUEBLO" (proposed name for Kiowa-
Tanoan, Keresan, and Zuni stocks)
QUORATEAN (see HOKAN)
Karok
SALISHAN
Chehalis
Clallam
Coeur d'Alene (or Skitswish)
Flathead (some of them)
Kalispel (or Pend d'Oreilles)
Lummi
Nisqually (or Nisqualli)
Nooksack (or Nooksak)
Puyallup
Quinaielt (or Quinault)

Salishan
Skagit
Skokomish
Snoqualmie (or Snoquamish)
Snohomish
Spokan
Suquamish (or Squawmish)
Swinomish
SHAHAPTIAN (linguistically related to
the Shapwailutan)
Nez Perce
Umatilla
Wallawalla
Warm Springs (or Tenino)
Yakima
SHAPWAILUTAN
Cayuse
Klamath
Modoc
SHOSHONEAN (see UTO-AZTECAN)
Bannock
Chemehuevi
Comanche
Goshute (or Gosiute)
Hopi
Paiute
Shoshone
Ute
SIOUAN
Assiniboin
Blackfoot (some of them)
Catawba
Crow
Dakota
Hidatsa
Iowa
Kaw (or Kansa)
Mandan
Omaha
Osage
Oto-Missouri
Ponca
Quapaw
Sioux
Winnebago
SKITTAGETAN
Haida
TONKAWAN
Tonkawa
UTO-AZTECAN (proposed name for
Piman and Shoshonean stocks)
WAKASHAN
Makah

Nootka
WASHOAN
Washoe
YUMAN (see HOKAN)
 Cocopah
 Havasupai
 Maricopa
 Mohave (or Mojave)
 Tonto

Walapai (or Hualapai)
Yavapai
Yuman
YUROK (or Weitspekan) (linguisti-
 cally related to Algonquin)
Yurok

ZUNI (see "PUEBLO")
Zuni